Books by James B. Maas

Power Sleep
(New York: HarperCollins, 1999)

Remmy and the Brain Train
(Ithaca, NY: Maas Presentations, 2001)

SLEEP
for
SUCCESS!

Everything You Must Know About Sleep but Are too Tired to Ask

Dr. James B. Maas
Rebecca S. Robbins
Cornell University

with Sharon R. Driscoll, Hannah R. Appelbaum, *and* Samantha L. Platt

authorHOUSE®

AuthorHouse™
1663 Liberty Drive
Bloomington, IN 47403
www.authorhouse.com
Phone: 1-800-839-8640

First published by AuthorHouse 1/25/2011

ISBN: 978-1-4520-3775-2 (sc)
ISBN: 978-1-4520-3776-9 (dj)
ISBN: 978-1-4520-3777-6 (e)

Library of Congress Control Number: 2010912304

Printed in the United States of America

This book is printed on acid-free paper.

Before making any changes in prescribed health-care regimens, make sure you consult
a licensed physician. While this book provides information on sleep strategies and
disorders, it is not intended to be a substitute for appropriate medical diagnosis or
treatment. If you are having a persistent problem, consult your physician and/or one of
the accredited sleep disorders centers listed on the internet at www.sleepcenters.org.

Dedicated to:

To Nancy, Dan and Justin Maas, and Martha, Todd, Mary and Will Robbins, whose love, support, patience and encouragement continue to make possible our journey towards enriching lives through sleep education.

J.B.M. R.S.R.

Contents

Acknowledgements

"Sleep for Success!" is based on the empirical research of dedicated sleep researchers who in the last decade have advanced our knowledge of sleep more than in all of past history. Wherever possible we have tried to give credit to specific individuals for key findings. However, the community of sleep researchers is a closely knit group who share ideas and discoveries openly, working cooperatively to solve the mysteries of the night. More often than not, the sleep advice in this book is based on the shared insights of several investigators whose primary motivation is not self-advancement, but rather the betterment of the human condition. If this book is helpful, it is due to the selfless and collective wisdom of the entire sleep profession.

There are individuals to whom we are profoundly indebted. For forty years Bill Dement, the Lowell W. and Josephine Q. Berry Professor of Psychiatry at Stanford University, has shared his insights on sleep research and his missionary zeal for informing the world about the central role of sleep in all human endeavors. He has guided us through the maze of the night and shed light on sleep's critical relevance to the day. He is a mentor and close friend. He introduced us to fellow sleep researchers Michel Jouvet, Thomas Roth, Charles Czeisler, Mary Carskadon, David Dinges, Curt Graeber, Mark Rosekind, Richard Ferber, Roslind Cartwright, Christian Guilleminault, Roger Broughton, J. Allan Hobson, Elliot Weitzman, Helene Porte, Milton Kramer, Michael Thorpy, John Lauber, Cheryl Spinweber, Carlos Schenck, Mark Mahowald, Jodi Mindell, Craig Boss, Sharon Smorch, and Martin Moore-Ede. Their pioneering work has been the focus of our films and presentations.

We are grateful for the editorial assistance of our dear friend and colleague, Joe Kita. His constructive criticism, creative voice, professionalism, sense of humor and ability to explain complex scientific concepts in readily accessible language were invaluable in helping us write *Sleep for Success!* We also are sincerely grateful for, and honored to have had the opportunity to work with, an incredibly skilled and talented team of research assistants. We extend our thanks to Hannah Appelbaum who contributed valuable research and insight in the early planning stages for *Sleep for Success!* and in particular for her work on the chapter, "What's Your Naptitude?" Sharon Driscoll contributed heavily to background research throughout the book and in particular to the segment on the bedroom environment in our chapter, "Sure Fire Strategies to Sleep for Success!" Sharon managed the meticulous task of editorial assistant, patiently formatting the manuscript umpteen times, and consistently supplying the enthusiasm and talent necessary to keep us on task. Her lunchtime piano concerts made long days of stressful editing for our staff much more bearable. Samantha Platt assumed the enormous task of collecting the many illustrations throughout the book (with the assistance of Zoe Proom), organized the obtaining of copyright permissions, and contributed background information for "The Architecture of a Good Night's Sleep."

We would like to express our appreciation to those individuals who did monumental background research and writing for specific chapters in "Sleep for Success!": Katie Hancock for Sleep from Birth through Childhood and Managing Time for Better Sleep; Maura Greenwood for Sleep and Drugs; Eve Burrough for Women and Sleep and Understanding and Treating the Most Common Sleep Disorders; Rebecca Fortgang for Surviving Shift Work; Liza Truax for Sleep, Exercise and the Athlete; and Andrew Bekkevold for Sleep Tips for the Traveler. We would like to recognize Nancy Haff of Williams College and Kate Riopelle of Michigan State University for doing background work on the science of sleep. Thanks are also due to Janet Maas Robinson, Roger and Caren Weiss, Enid and Jerry Alpern, Nancy and Nelson Schaenen, Jr., David Feldshuh, Bruce Levitt, Stephen Rogers, Phil Lempert, Dirk Dugan, Jon Mauser, Adam Law, Paul Hart, Ken Blanchard, Fisk Johnson, David Myers, Margarita Curtis, Peter Warsaw, Stuart Bicknell, Toby Emerson, William Robbins, Dave Dickinson, Derek Haswell, Don Hoffman, Ed McLaughlin, Brandon Palmer, Robert Hickman, Tracy Miller, Larry Pederson, Carolyn Levitan, Kristina Bisset, Sarah Hughes, Caroline Dupuis, Bobbie Molter, Andy Noel, Mike Schafer, Steve Donahue, John Melody, Steve Mountain, Lacey Flatt, Rosemary Avery, Lisa Proper, Pam Cunningham, Caroline Scott, Laura Justice, Rob Koll, Nathalie Weiss, Zoe Proom, Kali Gove, Megan Wherry Menner, Rebecca Dewitt, Greg Carroll, Thomas Gilovich, Jameer Nelson and the Orlando Magic for support and encouragement. And to Dr. Craig Boss and his staff (Sharon Smorch, Mae Hilliker, Shawn Webster and Nancy White) in Michigan at the Charlevoix Area Hospital Sleep Center, for scheduling internship sessions with our book researchers. In all our writing endeavors we have had the fortune of working closely with our office manager, Cindy Durbin, whose patience, understanding and hard work enabled us to teach, produce films, consult, fulfill speaking engagements and write with a minimum of distraction. Our sincerest thanks to Alan Bower, Lauren Allen, Sara Kelly and Hilary Jerrells of AuthorHouse who took this book under their wing, challenged us to shape it for maximum understanding and benefit, and made its publication feasible. Grace McQuade of the Goldberg-McDuffie Communications public relations agency put our *Power Sleep* book on the international media map and we are grateful that she will do the same for *Sleep for Success!*

We are deeply appreciative to the thousands of students at Cornell University in Ithaca, NY and the Weill Cornell Medical College in Doha, Qatar, as well as the corporate executives and professional athletes who have responded to our films, lectures and training seminars with enthusiasm and have challenged us to provide meaningful information to improve their alertness, success in life and well-being.

FOREWORD

William C. Dement, M.D., Ph.D.

Lowell W. and Josephine Q. Berry Professor of Psychiatry and Behavioral Science
School of Medicine, Stanford University
Chairman, National Commission on Sleep Disorders Research
Founder and former Director, Sleep Disorders Center

My relationship with Professor James Maas goes back a long way. We first worked together in 1968 when he approached me to participate in a film on sleep. If we complain today about the low level of public awareness regarding sleep knowledge, imagine what it was more than 40 years ago. Jim could probably, quite rightly, be labeled the world's first true sleep educator. Since that time, I have been privileged to appear in four subsequent films.

Although Professor Maas has carried out many other unrelated projects, the sleep field captured a major share of his enthusiasm and professional interest. I am sure that making an educational documentary on any subject is about as effective a learning experience as anyone can have. Soon, Jim was incorporating sleep material into his introductory psychology classes. As a result, more undergraduates were being exposed to the important facts of sleep each year at Cornell than all the rest of the world's undergraduates put together. His course regularly attracts 1,500-2,000 students and now he has taught the psychology of sleep to more than 65,000 undergraduates (and hundreds of Fortune 500 companies). Only a truly gifted educator could make such a large class simultaneously popular, rigorous and effective.

In "Sleep for Success" Professor Maas (and his colleague Rebecca Robbins) have focused their vast experience, expertise and educational talents in yet another educational venue. This effort, like the others, has the earmarks of a Jim Maas product: well organized, to the point, entertaining, and extremely well presented, indeed ingeniously presented.

Although I believe there should be effective education and enhanced awareness about the crucial facts of sleep in every component of society, it is clear that some initial focus is desirable if this gigantic challenge is to be met. My two choices for the highest priority public awareness targets are (a) those individuals whose work requires peak mental performance and creativity, and (b) those whose work performance can effect the safety of people and the environment. The most typical example of the latter is falling asleep at the wheel. Certainly this book should be read by everyone, but it is likely to be of greatest interest to high performance individuals, executives, managers, students, athletes, etc. where the rewards of achieving an optimal management of sleep should be achieved and the rewards will be great.

W.C.D.

Introduction

What's So "Macho" About Not Sleeping?

Unfortunately, most of us don't value sleep because we're blissfully ignorant of what can happen when we don't get enough of it. Many people regard sleep as a luxury, a waste of time, and even a weakness of character. How often have you heard the macho expression, "What do you mean you need eight hours of sleep, you sloth? Look at me, all I need is six!"

It's time we put an end to these myths and misplaced values. New research shows *we must stop resisting a rest.* We now know that quality sleep is an absolute necessity, and the sad and alarming truth is that the majority of the world's population doesn't get enough of it. Being truly sleep-deprived is different from being a little fatigued. If you're tired for 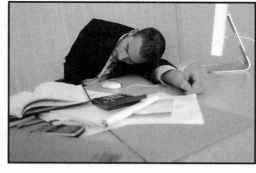 much of the day, then you have a serious pathological problem. Keep in mind that chronically sleepy people are the worst judges of their condition. They're often unaware of how significantly the lack of sleep affects mood, performance, relationships, health, and even longevity. In fact, sleep deprivation has probably been a major contributing factor to our many personal and collective misfortunes.

Sixty-five percent of us will have trouble falling asleep tonight and be exhausted tomorrow. Some of these tired people hold jobs that require alertness and quick decision-making. Sleep deprivation costs the United States alone *$66 billion* annually in lost productivity, accidents, illness, and premature death. It's making America unhealthy, stupid, clumsy, and perhaps even less respected and influential as a world leader.

Recent research has found a significant link between lack of sleep and stress, depression, ability to think and perform, hypertension, heart attacks, strokes, Type II diabetes, periodontal disease, skin problems, obesity, and cancer.

Fifty to seventy million people in the United States suffer from chronic sleep loss or sleep disorders. What's more, the US National Highway Traffic Safety Administration (NHTSA) estimates that drowsiness and/or fatigue is responsible for approximately 80,000 car accidents *per day* in America. These crashes result in an estimated 1,500 fatalities and 71,000 injuries each year for an annual loss of around $12.5 billion—all the result of something *preventable.*

It's time we learned to value sleep not as a luxury but as a necessity. Ignorance about its importance is no longer acceptable, nor is the veneration of those workaholics who disdain it. In this high-pressure world, we're obligated more than ever to know the facts and dangers. If we want to raise performance, reduce illness, improve general satisfaction with life and increase lifespan, we must pay attention to sleep as a fundamental biological process. "Encouraging a culture of sleepless machismo is worse than nonsensical; it is downright dangerous and the antithesis of intelligent management" (Harvard Business Review).

> New research shows that sleeping better is one of the simplest and most effective things we can do to vastly enhance and extend our lives.

There are ways to get great sleep, even if you've been experiencing insomnia or have one or more of the other eighty-nine known sleep disorders. Do you want to be healthier, more energetic, creative, organized, efficient, and constantly expanding your potential? Do you want to be less stressed, happier, have a better relationship with yourself and others, and have a deeper sense of well-being? What if you could take a few small steps every day that would enable you to sleep better and eventually achieve all these things?

You can. In fact, it's easy.

The solutions are at hand. You're holding them. Read on and enjoy *Sleep for Success*!

New Sleep Gadgets and Gizmos

Throughout the book we provide ratings of devices designed to help you get better sleep (from 1—not worth the money, to 5—of great value). We'll show you everything from the world's first sleep-phase alarm clock to a device guaranteed to cure your snooze-bar addiction.

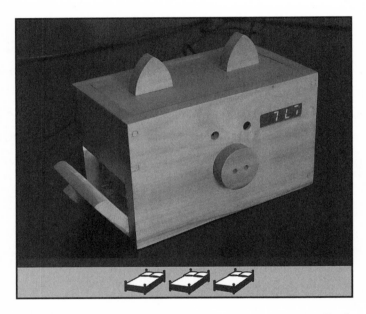

Wake 'n' Bacon Alarm Clock wakes you up to the smell of bacon.☺ Place frozen strips of bacon in the clock's chamber before going to bed. The bacon will be cooked before your alarm goes off so that you awake to a freshly cooked favorite breakfast item.

PART ONE

Everything You Must Know About Your Sleep Habits but Are Too Tired to Ask

1

The Sleep Meter: Think You're Alert? Find Out Here

- *Do you fall asleep as soon as your head hits the pillow?*
- *Do you need an alarm clock to wake up?*
- *Do you sleep extra hours on weekends?*

If you answered yes to these questions (and to others we're about to ask you), you're sleepier than you should be. You might feel alert enough to get through the day, but you're probably performing well below your potential.

Most people don't value sleep and have no idea how tired they really are. There are various elaborate and expensive laboratory tests that objectively measure sleepiness, but we can make a pretty thorough assessment based on how you respond to the following two questionnaires. Don't worry; they're short, easy, and fun—a cinch compared to any high school math exam.

The first self-test is the Maas Robbins Alertness Questionnaire (MRAQ). We've used this to assess Cornell University students as well as Fortune 500 executives. The twenty statements help differentiate between well-rested and sleep-deprived individuals. The second self test is the Epworth Sleepiness Scale. It measures daytime sleepiness and helps diagnose disorders such as sleep apnea and narcolepsy. Ready?

The Maas Robbins Alertness Questionnaire (MRAQ)

©2010 Dr. James B. Maas and Rebecca S. Robbins

Please indicate true or false for the following statements:

<u>True</u>   <u>False</u>

T   F   1. I often need an alarm clock in order to wake up at the appropriate time.

T   F   2. It's often a struggle for me to get out of bed in the morning.

T   F   3. Weekday mornings I often hit the snooze bar several times.

T   F   4. I often feel tired and stressed out during the week.

T   F   5. I often feel moody and irritable, and little things upset me.

T   F   6. I often have trouble concentrating and remembering.

T   F   7. I often feel slow with critical thinking, problem solving, and being creative.

T   F   8. I need caffeine to get going in the morning or make it through the afternoon.

T   F   9. I often wake up craving junk food, sugars, and carbohydrates.

T   F   10. I often fall asleep watching TV.

T   F   11. I often fall asleep in boring meetings or lectures or in warm rooms.

T   F   12. I often fall asleep after heavy meals or after a low dose of alcohol.

T   F   13. I often fall asleep while relaxing after dinner.

T   F   14. I often fall asleep within five minutes of getting into bed.

T   F   15. I often feel drowsy while driving.

T   F   16. I often sleep extra hours on the weekends.

T   F   17. I often need a nap to get through the day.

T   F   18. I have dark circles around my eyes.

T   F   19. I fall asleep easily when watching a movie

T   F   20. I rely on energy drinks or over-the-counter medications to keep me awake.

If you answered "True" to four or more of these statements, consider yourself seriously sleep-deprived.

Epworth Sleepiness Scale

(Designed by Dr. Murray Johns of Australia) ©M.W. Johns 1990–1997

Use the "Doze Scale" to respond to each situation.

0 = no chance of dozing
1 = slight chance of dozing
2 = moderate chance of dozing
3 = high chance of dozing

Situation	**Chance of Dozing**
Sitting and reading	_____
Watching TV	_____
Sitting inactive in a public place (theater/meeting)	_____
As a passenger in a car for an hour without break	_____
Lying down to rest in the afternoon when circumstances permit	_____
Sitting and talking to someone	_____
Sitting quietly after a lunch without alcohol	_____
In a car, while stopped for a few minutes in traffic	_____
MY Sleepy Score (Total Points)	_____

Results

If you scored …

Less than 8: Congratulations! You're getting adequate rest.

Between 8 and 11: You have mild sleepiness.

Between 12 and 15: You're moderately sleepy and must reevaluate your sleep habits.

Between 16 and 24: You're seriously sleep-deprived.

Before we discuss the serious, deleterious consequences of sleep deprivation and sleep disorders, take a moment to assess your sleep IQ by answering whether popular sleep beliefs are true or false:

Sleep Myths: What's Your Sleep IQ?

More myths exist about sleep than ancient Greece. This book separates fact from fable. Take the following quiz and see how much you know about sleep – something you should be spending one-third of your life doing *guiltlessly*.

Indicate true or false for the following statements:

True	False		
T	F	1.	Newborns dream less than adults.
T	F	2.	By playing audiotapes during the night, you can learn while you sleep.
T	F	3.	Chocolate candies on your hotel pillow help you sleep better.
T	F	4.	If you have insomnia, you should nap during the day.

T   F   5. Sleeping pills are helpful for people with long-term insomnia.

T   F   6. Your mattress doubles in weight every 10 years due to dead dust mites.

T   F   7. Sleep that begins before midnight is better than sleep that starts after midnight.

T   F   8. During sleep, the brain rests.

T   F   9. Sleeping longer can make you fat.

T   F   10. You can condition yourself to need less sleep.

T   F   11. Snoring isn't harmful as long as it doesn't disturb others.

T   F   12. The older you get, the fewer hours of sleep you need.

T   F   13. Most people realize when they're sleepy.

T   F   14. Drinking coffee, turning up the air-conditioning and cranking up the radio will help you stay awake while driving.

T   F   15. Sleep disorders are mainly due to worry or psychological problems.

T   F   16. The human body can never adjust to night-shift work.

T   F   17. Most sleep disorders go away without treatment.

T   F   18. If a smoke detector is as loud as a jet engine, a police siren or the Rolling Stones in concert, it will awaken your sleeping child.

T   F   19. People who sleep 6 hours or less are unlikely to improve athletic skills.

T   F   20. Grades would be higher, alertness would be greater, and discipline problems fewer, if high schools began classes after nine in the morning.

Questions 1-5, 7-15 and 17-18 are false. 6, 16, 19 and 20 are true. If you score poorly, don't worry; you already have all the correct answers in your hands. Just read on. *Sleep for Success!* is designed to provide clear explanations and practical solutions for all your sleep issues.

2

New Findings on Sleep Deprivation: The Silent Killer

So maybe you nod off in meetings every now and then, doing the old head-bob-I'm-awake-boss! dance. Or perhaps your mind wanders when you're driving, sometimes to the point that you can't recall how you got to your destination. Or maybe you're so tired during the day that your monthly Starbucks outlay now rivals your utilities bill—and, frankly, is just as necessary.

But do you have a problem? How much of this debilitating state is the result of leading a busy life in today's rather frenetic, 24/7 world? It's a similar question that people who drink alcohol occasionally ask themselves: Am I flirting with something dangerous here, a condition for which I need help?

Chances are if you're wondering about this then, yes, you do have a problem with sleep deprivation. To find out for sure, let's explore all the facets of this sneaky and debilitating disease. And it is a disease. In fact, if it were an option on death certificates, it could be checked off as the source of many an untimely demise.

Scared? Good!

What does it mean to be "sleep-deprived"?

You are sleep-deprived if you're not meeting your personal sleep need, which for most adults is between 7.5 and 9 hours per night. You should feel energetic, wide awake, and alert all day, without a significant midday drop in alertness. And the term "sleep-deprived" certainly applies to anyone who has difficulty falling asleep or staying asleep, wakes up too early, and/or has poor sleep quality.

Most Americans are at least modestly sleep-deprived. While the average person claims to get 7.1 hours of sleep per night, a study at the University of Chicago demonstrated that it's actually much less. Researchers attached small sleep-monitoring devices to subjects and found that those claiming 7 to 8 hours per night really slept closer to 6. It seems we're *so* sleep-deprived, we aren't even aware of how little we rest. And you can imagine what this means for the 55 percent of Americans who *think* they're getting 6 to 7 hours of sleep.

Who is sleep-deprived?

Most of us are moderately sleep-deprived; not just tired, but *deprived* of the very rest that is integral to health and competency in waking life. Pilots, doctors, nurses, teachers, students, politicians, executives, truck drivers, store clerks … all are veritable zombies. In general, high school and college students are the most pathologically sleep-deprived segment of the population. Their alertness during the day is on par with that of untreated narcoleptics and those with untreated sleep apnea. Not surprisingly, teens are also 71 percent more likely to drive drowsy and/or fall asleep at the wheel compared to

> ***President Bill Clinton:*** "You have no idea how many Republican and Democratic members of the House and Senate are chronically sleep-deprived. It makes them more edgy, it makes them more irritable, it makes them more vulnerable to being pulled back and forth by interest groups … sleep deprivation has a lot to do with some of the edginess in Washington today."

other age groups. (Males under the age of twenty-six are particularly at risk.)

Senior citizens and those in business and government are the next biggest group of yawners, with huge dips in alertness between 2:00 and 4:00 PM. Many of them brag about needing only five hours of sleep per night. Little do they know that it's undermining their job performance, putting them at risk for health problems, and even shortening their lives.

What are the signs of sleep deprivation?

Predictably, the most common symptom is fatigue. But as obvious as that seems, many people become so accustomed to feeling chronically tired that they accept it as normal. This same attitude is often applied to other symptoms such as mood swings, irritability, anxiety, and difficulty concentrating, remembering, learning, and interacting socially. You may feel you're a loner, a slow-learner, or just not a vibrant or ambitious person, when in fact your

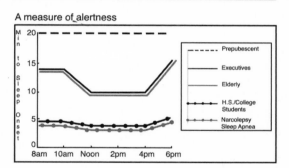

Fig. 1 indicates how quickly each group fell asleep when asked to try to fall asleep at six different time intervals throughout the day. It should take twenty minutes to fall asleep when fully rested.

fatigue has created a shell around your true personality and abilities. People don't recognize that sleepiness is not "normal," and something must be done to break the cycle.

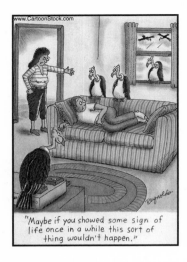

"Maybe if you showed some sign of life once in a while this sort of thing wouldn't happen."

Signs of chronic sleep deprivation can also include frequent infections/illnesses, blurred vision, changes in appetite, and depression. While these symptoms may be relatively minor and seem unrelated at first, they can be the precursors of life-shortening afflictions. Without proper treatment, they can grow to negatively impact your health and quality of life.

How do I know if I'm sleep-deprived?

The most thorough and reliable way to determine if you have a problem is to take a Multiple Sleep Latency Test (MSLT). The theory behind this test is that the faster you can fall asleep (when given the opportunity to do so in a quiet, dark, cool bedroom at specified intervals throughout the day), the more sleep-deprived you are. This test should be administered at an accredited sleep disorder center. You can visit www.sleepcenters.org to find the sleep lab nearest you.

> *Six Biggest Sleep Thieves:*
> - Alcohol or caffeine after 2 pm
> - Tobacco
> - Strenuous exercise within three hours of bedtime
> - A heavy meal within three hours of bedtime
> - A poor bedroom environment
> - Stress

What are the most common causes of sleep deprivation?

The biggest and most prevalent cause is our society's persistent belief that sleep is a luxury rather than a necessity. When it seems there just aren't enough hours in the day, sleep is the first thing we cut, though ironically if we slept more, we'd be more efficient and productive. The advent of the Internet, buzzing Blackberrys, and 24/7 entertainment has compounded the problem. Abusing sleep with blissful machismo is now deeply engrained in our global society.

Beyond this general notion, there are many specific contributing factors to sleep deprivation. *Temporary sleep loss*, for instance, is often triggered by passing stressors, such as a headache, toothache, indigestion, back problems, cold, flu, or jetlag. While these causes are certainly real and frustrating, they're relatively easy to treat.

> "Why sleep? I might miss a party. I'll sleep when I am dead."
> —*Janis Joplin, who died of a drug overdose at twenty-seven*

Anxiety is the most common cause of *short-term sleep loss*, and it can last for weeks. Nervousness about money, your marriage or relationship, losing or finding a job, your weight or other health concerns, and even boredom can all make you toss and turn.

Long-term sleep loss is occasionally caused by environmental factors—your job, if you're a night-shift worker; where you live, if it's in a noisy area—but it more commonly stems from medical conditions such as arthritis, diabetes, epilepsy, ulcers, and heart disease (among others), as well as consistent drug (including caffeine) or alcohol use. There are also a number of sleep-specific medical conditions that can severely impact and disrupt rest. These include sleep apnea, narcolepsy, restless leg syndrome, and upwards of eighty-six other distinguishable disorders, many of which are discussed in Chapter 17.

More than a third of people who suffer from chronic insomnia also have psychiatric conditions such as depression and schizophrenia, as well as obsessive-compulsive disorder, anxieties, or phobias. Sleep and psychiatric problems tend to go hand-in-hand—when you're not sleeping well, life appears grimmer; when life appears grim, it's harder to rest. Trouble sleeping can even be an early sign of forthcoming psychiatric problems, so it's important to talk to a doctor if symptoms arise or persist. For most patients, when an underlying mental condition is treated, sleep habits improve.

Does sleep deprivation affect me physically or behaviorally?

It affects you both ways. There's no escaping the debilitating effects of insidious sleepiness, no matter how motivated, responsible, or strong you are. Even in risky or potentially

> "You don't realize how fatigued you can be. I went to sleep one time in the Marine Corps—walking—and I walked about a mile, as best I can recall, until I fell into a ditch."
> —*Fred Smith, founder and chairman of the board, Federal Express*

dangerous situations, nothing can override the powerful and inevitable results of extensive or cumulative sleep loss. If you think you're in good shape but aren't sleeping well, you're cheating yourself out of an even better sense of well-being, little to no extra effort required.

Physical effects

Not sleeping makes you prone to:

- **Daytime drowsiness.** This usually manifests itself as a temporary drop in energy and alertness around mid-afternoon. It's accompanied by feelings of inattentiveness and grogginess, particularly when doing dull or repetitive tasks. It's more likely to occur after a heavy meal or a low dose of alcohol, or while sitting in a warm room, listening to a boring lecture, or participating in a dull meeting. These factors do not cause sleepiness; they simply unmask the physiological fatigue that's already present.

- **Microsleeps.** These are brief episodes of sleep that you're unaware of and that occur during waking hours. Lasting only a few seconds, microsleeps can produce inattention, resulting in accidents and injury.

- **Sleep seizures.** These are unintended longer episodes of sleep that come on as rapidly as a seizure, occurring without warning in a severely sleep-deprived person.

- **Colds and flu.** Dr. Jan Born at the University of Luebeck in Germany found that people who sleep less than six hours per night have 50 percent less resistance to viral infection than those getting eight hours of sleep. In addition, Dr. Sheldon Cohen of Carnegie Mellon University found that those sleeping less than seven hours per night are three times more likely to get a cold than longer-sleepers.

- **Weight gain.** You might think that spending more time in bed makes you lazy, but *not* spending enough time in bed can also make you fat. Lack of sleep lowers leptin levels in the brain and raises ghrelin levels in the stomach. These hormones are responsible for appetite regulation. So when you're sleep-deprived, you're more likely to overeat—craving carbs, sugars, and junk food.

   Researchers at Columbia University as well as the University of Chicago have found people who sleep five hours per night have a 50 percent higher chance of being obese, while those who sleep six hours have a 23 percent greater risk.

   Professor Francesco Cappuccio at the University of Warwick Medical School found that less sleep is associated with an almost two-fold increase in obesity—a trend that he says is detectable in children as young as five. The research also linked short sleep with a higher body-mass index (BMI) and waist circumference over time.

- **Diabetes.** A study at the University of Chicago involving healthy young men with no risk factor for diabetes found that after just one week of inadequate sleep, they were in a pre-diabetic state. Researchers attributed the result to overactive central nervous systems (caused by not sleeping), which affected the ability of the pancreas to produce enough insulin to adequately regulate glucose levels. The current epidemic in diabetes may be connected to the epidemic in sleep deprivation. We now have an epidemic of early onset childhood diabetes, and it appears to be linked to obesity and lack of sleep.

> *Sleep More, Drop Blood Pressure:* One extra hour of sleep per night decreases the risk of artery calcification by 33 percent. Plus, it's accompanied by a 17-mm drop in systolic blood pressure.
> —*Dr. Diane Lauderdale, University of Chicago*

- **Heart disease.** Not sleeping often causes the body to produce more stress hormones. Such an imbalance can lead to arteriosclerosis, which can cause heart attacks and strokes, in addition to hypertension, muscle loss, increased fat storage, loss of bone mass, and lower production of growth hormone and testosterone.

  In addition, short-sleepers miss out on REM sleep (predominant between the seventh and eighth hours of the night), during which time the heart pumps more blood to the muscles. This helps it relax as blood pressure falls. So, by cutting back on sleep, we're preventing this innate regulating system from doing its job. Additionally, sleep apnea, if undiagnosed and/or untreated, significantly raises the risk of cardiovascular disease because the heart must work harder to oxygenate the blood.

- **Cancer.** Women who exercise regularly and were generally healthy had a 47 percent higher risk of cancer if they were sleeping fewer than seven hours. Researchers at Stanford University also found that good sleep habits can be a valuable weapon in fighting cancers, citing melatonin (released during sleep) and cortisol production (involved in regulating immune system activity) as vital players in patient recovery.

Night-shift workers (both male and female) have a 35 percent higher risk of colorectal cancer. Why? According to the International Agency for Research on Cancer, shift-work is not a "possible" but a "probable" carcinogen, due to too much light exposure and lack of melatonin secretion in your brain because you are not sleeping.

Blind women have 50 percent less chance of breast cancer than sighted women. Why? Active, sighted women often stay up late, spending too much time in the light. Again, exposure to light and lack of sleep block the release of cancer-fighting melatonin and raise estrogen levels, which can cause breast cancer.

People who sleep well and are less stressed during traumatic times in their life due to illnesses like cancer live longer and are less affected by their illness than those who get easily stressed by these big life changes. Additionally, therapies like yoga have been proven to help cancer patients (who are often affected with chronic insomnia) sleep better and therefore feel better.

- **Skin.** Sleep is essential for rebuilding tissues and cells, including the skin. Sufficient sleep is required to maintain good skin texture and a healthy glow. The first area of skin to be affected by a lack of sleep is the eyelids. The skin is very thin here so lack of sleep causes puffy eye bags, fine lines, and dark circles. In the long term, lack of sleep causes skin to age faster leading to wrinkles, poor texture, and discoloration much earlier in life than in the well-rested individual. During sleep, the body metabolizes free radicals, which accelerate aging and cancerous growths. Without sufficient sleep, there are more free radicals present in the skin leading to poor skin quality and even skin cancer. Sustained sleep deprivation impairs host defense so if the skin is exposed to bacteria or is healing from a lesion, lack of sleep will increase the amount of healing time required and may result in more severe bacterial skin infections.

- **Poor athletic performance.** Since sleepiness impairs reaction time, awareness, and motor skills, it should come as no surprise that well-rested athletes enjoy the best performance.

    During sleep, the brain moves short-term muscle memory (of a tennis serve, a basketball shot, or a golf swing that you've been practicing) into long-term muscle memory, where you can more easily retrieve it later. So the adage "practice makes perfect" only works if it's followed by adequate rest, meaning we should really be saying "practice with sleep makes perfect."

    In fact, research shows that athletes who forego early morning workouts to sleep in and train only in the afternoon are likely to perform better than those who do double sessions.

As you can see, if you thought that a little fatigue was the worst outcome of sleep deprivation, you were wrong.

Behavioral effects

Not sleeping makes you prone to:

- **Mood shifts, including depression and irritability.** Mood is one of the first traits to be affected by sleep loss. Miss even one night of sound rest and your threshold for anger lowers.

You can quickly lose friends, upset loved ones, foil negotiations, and make enemies.

- **Stress, anxiety, and loss of coping skills.** Sleep loss leads to amygdala activation, the area of your brain involved in rage and aggression. There's also decreased activity in your limbic system, which regulates anxiety. Feelings of not being able to cope, even with simple problems or moderate workloads, can become overwhelming and result in increased worry, frustration, and nervousness. You can lose your perspective and be unable to relax under even moderate pressure. Stress produces sleep loss, and sleep loss produces stress. It's a very vicious cycle. While the sleep-deprived are shuffling through life and have less control over emotions, the well-rested are more alert and less stressed.

> *A Fatal Mistake:*
>
> A five-month-old boy died of heat exhaustion after he was forgotten for nearly ten hours in the back seat of a car. His father, a computer programmer, was supposed to drop his son at day care at 7:30 am but forgot the baby was in the car and went to work. He didn't realize his mistake until 5:15 pm, when his wife went to the sitter, learned the baby was not there, and called her husband. According to the doctor who performed the autopsy, the boy appeared to have struggled furiously against his seat belt and died of extreme heat exhaustion and hyperthermia in the "enormously hot" car. Even after he had been dead for some time, the infant's temperature was 106 degrees. The father was described by a co-worker as "a dedicated, driven employee who put in a lot of extra hours, and had probably overworked himself that week to the point of distraction. He was overtired, I guess."

- **Socializing less.** In short, you'd rather stay home than go out. It's not because you're anti-social; it's just that you're too tired.

- **Sub-par mental functioning/perception.** Whether you realize it or not, losing sleep makes you less efficient at just about every task and, in general, creates a dulled-down version of yourself, with a duller reaction to negative events, and even a drop in your taste sensitivity.

- **Concentration problems.** Since your mental faculties are not alert, sleep loss affects focus.

- **Difficulties with memory** (especially short-term). Functional magnetic resonance imagery (FMRI) scans of brain activity in sleep-deprived individuals trying to perform even simple tasks show momentary lapses of functioning in several important regions. During sleep, the brain moves short-term muscle memory into long-term muscle memory, where you can more easily retrieve it later. It also affects your ability to think logically and critically, making it difficult to assimilate and analyze new information. When you're sleepy, your brain works in a completely different way from when it's well rested. In fact, some parts don't work much at all. FMRI images show that sleep-deprived brains have much less activity in the right hippocampus. Thus, losing sleep means losing memory, and not just for tomorrow- but for months afterwards.

- **Failing to analyze and assimilate new information.**

- **Reduced ability to communicate.** Speaking and writing skills deteriorate with sleep loss.

- **Lower creativity.** Lack of sleep severely disrupts many duties of the hippocampus, which means you'll have less ability to conceptualize.

- **Impaired motor skills and coordination.**

Would you hire a person with these characteristics? Next time you interview someone for a job, ask how many hours of sleep he or she gets per night. If it's six or less, call in the next candidate.

How does sleepiness affect my ability to drive?

Sleep deprivation dampens your senses and impairs your perception, much like driving drunk or under the influence of drugs. One drink of alcohol on six hours of sleep is the equivalent of six drinks on eight hours of sleep in terms of your ability to drive. Never get into a car with anyone who is the least bit sleep-deprived and has been drinking alcohol. Driving drowsy has the same effect as driving drunk. Perhaps police should augment the breathalyzer with a sleepalyzer.

How can I "cure" my sleep deprivation?

It's simple: sleep better and sleep more. Most people need to rest just one extra hour per night to stay completely alert all day. It'll take a few weeks to effectively change your schedule to accommodate this, but eventually you should be waking up naturally without an alarm clock. After just a few nights of meeting your personal sleep quotient by improving your sleep strategies, you should feel a notable difference.

How do you change? We'll explain all of that in great detail in the next few chapters. Once you fix your sleep habits, you'll *Sleep for Success!*, and you'll say what everyone else does: "I never knew what it was like to be awake."

PART TWO

New Discoveries in the Science of Sleep

3
The Architecture of a Good Night's Sleep

What goes on when the lights go off?

Given that we spend (or *should* spend) one-third of our lives sleeping, it's alarming how little we know about our downtime. Even most doctors are not fully informed because, until recently, sleep was rarely mentioned in medical school, much less included as a significant part of their professional education. Plus, doctors are extraordinarily sleep-deprived during their residency. As a result of it they make mistakes, sometimes fatal to their patients. Does it surprise you that 40 percent of laypersons and physicians think the brain shuts down and takes a rest when we fall asleep? In actuality, the sleeping brain is highly dynamic and, at times, even more active than when we're awake. The sleeping brain plays a dramatic role in maintaining and regulating cardiovascular, gastrointestinal, and immune functions. It also facilitates mental processes such as learning, memory, creativity, and problem-solving. And it is the repository of your dreams.

We don't expect you to become an expert in sleep mechanics, but the more you understand about it, the more likely you'll be to prioritize and improve your sleep habits. So here are the basics:

How do I know what happens when I sleep?

Imagine you've come to a state-of-the-art sleep lab. (Most of them now look like five-star hotels rather than scientific laboratories.) You've been hooked up to various devices that measure brainwaves, eye movements, muscle tension, body temperature, respiration, heart rate, and hormonal activity. You might feel like Medusa with all these wires hooked to your body. But trust us—you'll still be able to fall asleep. The technician will tuck you in and turn off the light, setting the stage for the theater of the night.

Many people believe that soon after going to bed they drift into deep sleep, remain there for some time, have an occasional dream, and then awaken for the new day. There are several stages of sleep, however, each marked by significant changes in all those things being monitored and more.

The night is basically divided into non-REM (non-rapid eye movement) and REM (rapid eye movement) sleep. REM sleep is the period in which most dreams take place. Non-REM is also referred to as "slow-wave" sleep and is subdivided into several stages, earmarked by different brainwaves and purposes.

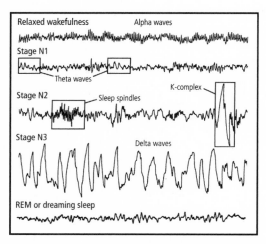

Fig. 2 Brain waves, detected by an electroencephalogram, record the stages of sleep. The "N" designates slow-wave or non-REM sleep. Stage N4 (not illustrated here) consists solely of delta waves.

So here's what really happens after you turn off Jay Leno, David Letterman, or Conan O'Brien. As you close your eyes, your brainwaves become slower and more regular. These alpha waves look like the teeth of a comb and signify a relaxed yet still wakeful state. This stage is akin to meditation. Next is the so-called Stage 1 period, when you have theta waves for about five minutes as your breathing slows. The large muscles begin to relax. The transition to Stage 2 is sometimes marked by a fleeting sensation of falling, causing you to wake momentarily with a jerk (not referring to your spouse). During this period, you disengage from the environment and become blissfully unaware of any outside stimuli. Researchers believe Stage 2 is the beginning of actual sleep. It's marked by spikes in brainwave activity called sleep spindles and K-complexes, which interrupt those previously regular waves. (As you'll see in Chapter 16, sleep spindles also play a significant role in athletic performance.) Stage 2 lasts ten to twenty-five minutes, but you'll return to it several times before daybreak, accounting for half of your night's slumber.

Next comes Stage 3 sleep, which is characterized by slow brainwaves called theta waves. These are interspersed with even slower delta waves. You'll spend just a half hour here, but eventually it will comprise up to 20 percent of your total night's sleep.

When the theta waves disappear, you enter Stage 4, the deepest sleep stage, which consists totally of delta waves. On your initial visit, it lasts for thirty to forty minutes. If aroused during Stage 4, you'll feel groggy and disoriented. During this stage, blood pressure drops, respiration slows, and blood flow to your muscles decreases. The secretion of growth hormone by the pituitary gland also peaks, stimulating body development and tissue repair. That's why uninterrupted deep sleep of significant duration is especially critical for children and adolescents. And it's also why we sleep more when we're sick. So, in Stage 4, you're completely out of it and at your most vulnerable. It's the closest humans get to hibernation.

When do I dream?

After thirty to forty minutes of Stage 4 sleep, you retrace your steps through Stages 3 and 2. You've now been asleep for about ninety to one hundred minutes. Then something astonishing happens. Instead of

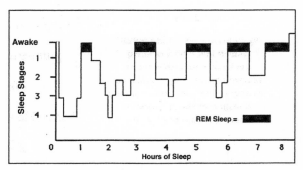

Fig. 3 shows the architecture of a good night's sleep. The dark blocks represent your time spent in REM sleep. Each REM cycle should be longer than the previous. Therefore, your sleep between hours seven and eight are critical for memory.

going back into Stage 1 or "twilight" sleep, your sympathetic nervous system becomes more active than it is in slow-wave sleep or even when awake. Blood flow to the brain, respiration, pulse rate, blood pressure, and body temperature all increase. Your eyes dart back and forth under their lids, and you enter the highly active stage of REM sleep.

Here, messages from the brain's motor cortex are blocked at the brainstem. As a result, muscles relax, and you're unable to move. That's why REM sleepers are described as having "an active brain in a paralyzed body." It's during the first part of REM that you experience your first dream of the night. Just like clockwork (because, in fact, this entire system

> *Honey, what the heck are you dreaming about?*
>
> During REM sleep, men often get penile erections and women experience clitoral erections, increased vaginal blood flow, and uterine contractions. This is typically unrelated to dream content or arousal and is quite normal.

is run by your biological clock), you enter REM sleep every ninety minutes throughout the night. When you're sleeping adequately, you visit it four to five times, with each REM period being twice as long as the last. This is why your final few hours of rest are so important; they're almost entirely REM sleep. If you're asleep for eight hours, you'll have spent between one and a half to two hours of the night in REM.

Although dreaming can occur in all stages, about 85 percent takes place here. REM dreams are usually the most vivid and emotional. But REM isn't just about dreaming. The previous day's events are solidified into permanent memory traces, and sequences of learned skills (like a new golf swing) become muscle memories.

4 Sleep, Learning, and Memory

Our ancient ancestors viewed sleep as a mysterious, inert state that somehow played a role in survival. For them, sleep also made practical sense as a way to recuperate from fatigue and avoid nighttime dangers (i.e., being eaten by predators or falling off cliffs). Researchers are just beginning to fully understand the complexities of our sleeping selves and the powerful resulting impact on our waking lives.

We sleep for two reasons: First, our bodies run on cycles called circadian rhythms, of which the sleep cycle is one. Many of these cycles, such as heartbeat, blood pressure, respiration, metabolism, and temperature, drop or slow during the sleep cycle. Mission control for all these processes is a part of the midbrain called the

> "If sleep has no purpose, it's the biggest mistake evolution ever made."
> —*Dr. Allan Rechtschaffen, a pioneer sleep researcher*

suprachiasmatic nucleus. This is where your master body clock is located. If this nucleus is damaged or removed, you end up taking lots of short naps instead of having one long sleep period.

Your circadian rhythms are set by various time cues called zeitgebers. Light is the most powerful cue affecting sleep. Daylight wakes you up, and darkness triggers the release of the hormone melatonin that brings on sleep. Noise and temperature can also play key roles in the regulation of your sleep schedule.

The second reason we sleep is that the longer we're awake, the greater our need for mentally and physically restorative sleep. It takes one hour of sleep to pay for every two hours of wakefulness. So, we start to tire after being up for about sixteen hours. Sleep debt is cumulative, which means the longer you deprive yourself of rest, the more of it you'll need to feel rested. How drowsy or alert you are depends on both your circadian rhythms and your sleep debt.

How much do I move around while I'm sleeping?

Everyone moves around somewhat during sleep, and these movements are coordinated with certain points in the sleep cycle. Even if you fall asleep and wake up in the same position, chances are you've tossed and turned as many as sixty times during the night. Movements often mark the transition periods between sleep stages. In fact, only in REM sleep is there no movement. Thus, we can dream about a midnight snack, but we won't be heading for the fridge anytime soon.

> *Synchronized Sleeping:* Couples who have been together a while move during sleep in a coordinated fashion, reducing the chances of bumping and waking each other.

Does experiencing all the sleep stages every night really matter?

To be wide awake, energetic, and psychologically, emotionally, and physiologically at your best, you must play every movement of the symphony of the night. The problem is many of us never get beyond stage 2 sleep due to stress, aging, or medications taken for other medical problems such as rheumatoid arthritis, hypertension, or Type II diabetes.

If you have trouble sleeping after taking a new medication, ask your doctor if there are alternative prescriptions.

How do I know if I am getting good deep and REM sleep?

In the past, going to a sleep lab for an expensive ($1500–$2,000), all-night sleep recording was the only way to get a good picture of your sleep patterns. Now there are devices you can use at home to give you a pretty good analysis of your sleep. One of the most accurate (and costs just $199), is the ZEO device.

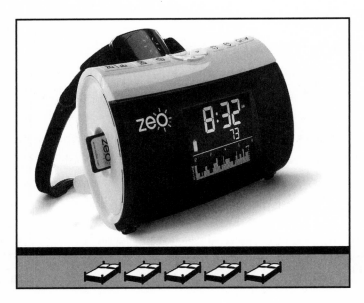

The Zeo Personal Sleep Coach is a science-based educational tool and motivational program that allows you to track your personal sleep patterns and reveal lifestyle habits and behaviors that may help or hinder your sleep. It also provides personalized coaching and advice to help you get a better night's rest. The device is composed of a headband, a bedside display, and a coaching program at myzeo.com.

The Zeo Headband sends your personal sleep information wirelessly to a bedside display, which provides a window into how you slept the previous night. It shows you an array of personal sleep information including:

Sleep Graph—summarizes sleep phase patterns each night.

ZQ—a single score created to help quickly gauge the quantity, quality, and depth of your sleep each night. ZQ can range from 0 to 120 or more depending on factors like age, gender, and stress level.

Total Z—how long you really slept the previous night, counting any perceived and unperceived awakenings that can be detected.

Time to Z—the time it took you to fall asleep.

Time in Wake & Times Woken.

Total amount of REM, Light, & Deep sleep.

By the way, we've heard of entire families that vie with each other for the highest Z score of the night.☺

What is sleep's role in learning, remembering, creating, and problem-solving?

Are you looking for a promotion? Trying to be more creative? Do you need to learn a new skill or solve an old problem? Having an excellent memory and sharper insight will help you realize all these things, and the way to develop them is with adequate sleep. Learning ability, memory consolidation, creativity, and problem-solving are all severely compromised by even a little sleep loss. New research shows that sleep

> *Say That Again*
>
> There is a 19 percent memory deficit in sleep-deprived individuals, meaning that most of us are operating at only 80 percent of our potential.

and mental functioning are closely linked. But we didn't need science to tell us that. Just look around at the successful, happy people you know. Are they the ones falling asleep at their desks, in meetings, or on the couch after dinner? To the contrary, those who are most productive and prosperous are the ones who are well rested (and who can remember what they had for dinner the previous night). No doubt about it, the best brain food is a good night's rest.

In almost every psychological experiment testing brain functioning, whether the test involves remembering pairs of words, tapping numbered keys in a certain order, or figuring out the rules in a weather-prediction game, "sleeping on it" after first learning the task improves performance. It's as if our brains squeeze in some extra practice time while we're asleep. Sleep also seems to be the time when the brain's two memory systems—the hippocampus and the neocortex—"talk" with one another.

Experiences that become memories are laid down in the hippocampus in the first two hours of sleep. In the next four hours, if a memory is to be retained it must be transferred from the hippocampus to a place where it will have physical permanence—the neocortex, the wrinkled outer layer of the brain where higher thinking takes place.

Stickhold and Wehrwein report, "Unlike the hippocampus, the neocortex is a master at weaving the old with the new. And partly because it keeps incoming information at bay, sleep is the best time for the 'undistracted' hippocampus to shuttle memories to the neocortex, and for the neocortex to link them to related memories." During the final two hours of REM sleep, the brain takes the information and repeatedly reruns it in a process called *REM replay*. So as you can see, any sleep longer than six hours helps in memory retention, but it takes eight hours to fully incorporate learned material. That's why you should make an extra effort to get a full night's sleep after studying for an exam, rehearsing a presentation, or learning a new set of skills.

> *Winning the Rat Race:* When rats are trained to run a maze, during that night's sleep their brains rehearse the proper turns. By recording activity in their motor cortex, scientists can tell the exact location in the maze that the rat's brain is rehearsing. This same sleep process helps you incorporate your tennis lessons or figure out the new software you're using at work.

Different sleep stages contribute to formation of different kinds of memory. Memories of personal experiences, called episodic memories, are formed during slow-wave sleep. Procedural memories, formed by learning a new skill, are consolidated during REM sleep.

What's the minimum amount of sleep I can get without my memory or learning being affected?

When it comes to memory, shortened sleep is bad news. No matter how intelligent you are, losing sleep means losing brain power. People who sleep less than six hours after learning new information show *no* improvement the next day, and those who don't sleep at all perform only half as well on memory tests as their well-rested counterparts.

> *Sleep is not something that can be put off until the weekend.*
> Get a good night's sleep every night, and you will see improvements in memory, attentiveness, and problem solving.

Here's another interesting ripple: In order to prepare information for retention, the brain filters out what's unimportant and solidifies the essentials, cross-referencing it with what's already on file. This process of making connections between the new information and what was previously known is called *memory consolidation*. With inadequate sleep, you may be able to *form* new memories, but you won't be able to *retain* them.

There is a direct correlation between REM sleep and learning efficiency. In fact, it seems the brain knows when it needs more consolidation time. Researchers studying people in intensive language programs have found that the amount of time they spend in REM sleep naturally increases the night after learning. As a result, they benefit from protein synthesis during REM sleep that increases the strength of the connections between brain cells and facilitates memory consolidation. (In other words, you should see these folks conjugate Arabic verbs!) During REM sleep, the brain is able to remove irrelevant details, creatively process the information, and even restore temporarily misplaced information that you couldn't recall during the day. This purging and purifying removes poor information that is competing with pertinent material, thereby enhancing memory.

Can I learn while I'm sleeping?

You can't acquire entirely new information while sleeping. So forget about trying to master a new language or expand your vocabulary through the night by listening to audiotapes. For the most part, any auditory information we receive during sleep goes in one ear and out the other, with no processing by the brain. Thus, you won't be able to recall a thing. However, during sleep you definitely rehearse and consolidate information acquired while you were awake. So if you're trying to learn new vocabulary or memorize a speech, review the material just before turning off the lights, and when you wake up in the morning you'll recall it better!

How much will losing an entire night of sleep hurt me?

It will have a profound impact. Physical movements will be sluggish, focusing will be difficult, and you'll tend to "zone out" more frequently.

Functional magnetic resonance imagery (FMRI) scans of brain activity in sleep-deprived individuals trying to perform even simple tasks show momentary lapses of functioning in several regions essential for cognitive processing.

Can sleep make me more creative?

Scientists, writers, and artists have made discoveries or had insights while sleeping that changed the world. If it wasn't for dreams, Mendeleev wouldn't have completed the periodic table, Singer wouldn't have invented the sewing machine, and the Nike brand name wouldn't exist.

Research shows that subjects who slept adequately were almost three times more likely to gain insight into a problem than those who remained awake. Are you struggling with a challenging project or dilemma? If so, the solution might lie in eight hours of sleep.

Is sleep more important before or after learning?

Both are crucial for memory retention. Loss of REM sleep prior to learning can result in a 50 percent reduction in the awareness of mental cues that help to establish memory. It also severely disrupts many duties of the hippocampus, which means you'll have less ability to conceptualize, a duller reaction to negative events, and even a drop in your taste sensitivity (the sensory kind, not your preference for Barry Manilow).

Adequate sleep after learning, however, is most crucial. This is the only time that memory enhancement occurs. Research subjects who were deprived of sleep the first night after learning still showed no sign of improvement even after two subsequent nights of full sleep. In some cases, it has even been shown that people develop amnesia for the information learned. The simple truth is if you're not sleeping after learning new information, you might as well spare yourself the trouble of learning in the first place. You need to remember to sleep because you have to sleep to remember!

> **Improve Your Pitch:**
> - Calling all singers! Sleep modifies brain activities involved in song production, allowing for improvement in pitch and tone.
> - Athletic performance Motor skills can increase 19 percent to 21 percent after just one night of improved sleep.

How is brain activity altered when I don't get enough sleep?

When you're sleepy, your brain works in a completely different way than when it's well rested. In fact, some parts don't work much at all. FMRI images show that sleep-deprived brains have much less activity in the right

> **Is your boss under the influence?**
> After seventeen to nineteen hours without sleep, brain activity is similar to someone with a Blood Alcohol Content (BAC) of 0.05 (0.08 is the legal limit for intoxication). Reaction time will also decline by 50 percent. After someone has been awake for twenty-eight hours, they'll be behaving as though they have a BAC of 0.1

hippocampus (memory center). Thus, losing sleep means losing memory, and not just for tomorrow—but for months afterwards.

So how do people manage to get by if parts of their brain aren't functioning normally?

Other brain areas pick up the slack. It's like hobbling around on crutches—arms aren't usually involved in walking, but when called upon for assistance they contribute more to the process. Altered functioning of the brain results in altered behavior, as though you have a sort of mental limp. You have lost effectiveness.

By comparison, people who have slept a full night show increased activity in the cerebellum, a region of the brain responsible for speed and accuracy. There's also decreased activity in their limbic system, which regulates anxiety. Yet with sleep loss, the amygdala, an area of your brain involved in rage and aggression, becomes more activated. So while the sleep-deprived are shuffling through life and have less control over their emotions, the well rested are more alert and less stressed.

5 Dreaming

How much do we dream?

If you sleep for eight hours, you'll dream three to five times, spending about one hundred minutes in your theater of the night. Dreams, which occur about every ninety minutes during sleep, typically last from nine minutes to as long as thirty minutes or more. They may include visual imagery and sensations of taste, smell, hearing, or pain. They range from the realistic and easily understood to the illogical and incomprehensible. Sometimes our dreams seek gratification of personal wishes, which are often socially unacceptable desires that are aggressive and/or sexual in nature. They're often based on daytime experiences and can reveal fears, frustrations, or even attempts to prophesize future events. They can be in color or black-and-white; it doesn't matter as far as dream content.

People who are extroverted seem to remember more of their dreams than those who tend to be more guarded and introverted. Most of the dreams we do remember are the last ones we had just prior to awakening. The interpretation and meaning of dreams has been debated throughout the centuries, and scientists are still working to shed light on their origin, purpose, and meaning.

What are the various types of dreams?

Prophetic Dreams or Precognitive Dreams

These are dreams that are believed to signify future events. Hungarian Bishop Joseph Lanyi dreamt of the assassination of Archduke Ferdinand in 1914. He wrote down and drew everything as he'd seen it in his dream, and it bore an uncanny resemblance to what happened several days later. President Abraham Lincoln dreamt that he heard subdued sobs, as if a number of people were weeping in the White House. He wandered into the East Room and saw a coffin lying on a platform; the face of the deceased was covered. When Lincoln demanded who was in the coffin, one of the soldiers guarding the body said, "The President. He's been killed by an assassin!" Two weeks later, Lincoln unfortunately met a similar fate. Perhaps chance and educational guesses are at work? As intriguing and compelling as such "accurate" dream predictions are, there are many more "prophetic" dreams that do not come true and therefore receive no attention.

Cultural events have often taken place because a dreamer decided to undertake a project or pursue a goal based on inspiration from a dream. Harriet Tubman claimed that her dreams helped her find safe pathways for the Underground Railroad, which served as the route to freedom for many slaves. Mohandas Gandhi had a dream of people in India stopping their businesses for twenty-four hours, which resulted in the nonviolent strikes in 1919. They marked a turning point in India's efforts to achieve self-determination. Lyndon Johnson had a dream that shifted his outlook during the Vietnam conflict. He dreamt he was in the middle of a river, and despite his attempts, was going around in circles. He shortly thereafter announced his intention to not run for another term.

Recurrent Dreams

Approximately two thirds of adults experience repetitive, often disturbing, dreams. These are sometimes modified over time and become more pleasant, especially if an underlying disturbance has been resolved in real life.

Nightmares vs. Night Terrors

REM anxiety dreams (bad dreams) are what most people think of as nightmares. But this is quite different from night terrors, a sleep disorder accompanied by screaming and moaning. Night terrors usually occur within the first two hours of sleep, often as an arousal from Stage 4 deep sleep. Pulse and blood pressure rise rapidly, but as frightening as they are to an observer, there is generally no recall of the event by the sleeper.

Lucid Dreams

Lucid dreaming is being aware that you are dreaming while you're in the process of having a dream. People who are capable of lucid dreaming can control and remember their dreams as clearly as if they were awake. Like normal dreaming, it usually takes place during REM sleep. Theoretically, we all have the capacity to have lucid dreams and influence their outcome, although it takes considerable time and effort to learn how to do it successfully. If you're interested, read *Lucid Dreaming: A Concise Guide to Awakening in Your Dreams and in Your Life*, by Stanford expert Stephen LaBerge. Tibetan Buddhists have been practicing dream yoga, very similar to Western lucid dreaming, for thousands of years.

Are dreams influenced by daytime experiences?

Dreams often seem to be stimulated by what happens to us during our waking hours. They are often considered "day residue," playing out situations and feelings left over from the previous day. Dream researcher

Rosalind Cartwright says that if you fall asleep thinking about something disappointing, your brain takes that information and lays it over

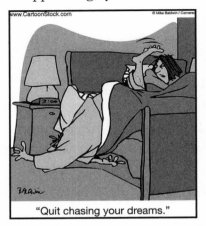

"Quit chasing your dreams."

experiences that are somehow matches in the "same emotional network of memory." This is how a bad day can translate into a bad dream. During the night, with each passing REM stage, the plots of dreams get more intricate and include older images that are increasingly distant from current reality. By morning, your dreams are more pleasant if, by the last REM period, your brain has found matches in old memories that are associated with the same initial bad feeling but had a good outcome.

Odors can influence the emotional content of your dreams. Pleasant smells, like roses, caused sleeping volunteers to experience pleasant emotions in their dreams. Negative smells, like rotten eggs, caused the same volunteers to experience negative emotions while dreaming.

How can I interpret my dreams? (Or should I even bother?)

Uncovering the source or meaning of dreams is difficult to do in any scientific way. So what's the most modern theory about the origin of dreams? Professor J. Alan Hobson and Robert W. McCarley of Harvard Medical School hypothesize that the content of dreams may well be meaningful, but many aspects of dreaming previously believed to be psychologically important are, in fact, simple reflections of physiological changes in the brain. Hobson and McCarley feel that dreaming is an unimportant byproduct of random neuronal activity. Their activation-synthesis hypothesis asserts that the firing of nerve cells in the lower brain stem during REM sleep randomly activates parts of the cerebral cortex that hold ideas and memories. Our brain tries to make sense of the neural activity by synthesizing the impulses into what we experience as dreams. The synthesis may involve unresolved daytime issues, but it could just as well be a compilation of memories triggered at random. Maybe that's why we sometimes dream of people interacting who would never be together in "real life." The fact that newborns and many lower species also spend considerable time in REM sleep lends credence to the theory that not all dreams are the result of unsettled personal events or the need to gratify basic desires. Maybe they're just memory traces activated at random by lower brain centers that are working the night shift.

Whatever you think about dreams, it is fun (and maybe even helpful) to take the time to think about why you might have had certain scripts played out in your theater of the night. Do your dreams have literal meaning, or do they represent meaningless manifest content? (What associations come to mind when you review your dream content? Is the policeman in your dreams just a policeman, or is he a disguised symbol of your authoritarian father? Is a cigar just a cigar, or is it a symbol for a penis? Even Freud admitted sometimes a cigar is just a cigar!) Do your dreams represent desires wishing for gratification? Is it all just nonsense? Or do your dreams illuminate issues worthy of daytime consideration? You be the judge.

PART Three

A New Look on How to Get a Great Eight Hours of Sleep

6
The Four Essential Keys to Sleeping Well

Optimal Sleep for Optimal Living

We know most of you don't value sleep. You consider it a luxury rather than a necessity and, as a result, you aren't willing to adjust your schedule to get adequate rest. But give us one week. That's all we ask. Follow our four simple keys for seven days, and you'll experience—perhaps for the first time since you were a child—what it feels like to be fully awake. More sleep means better daytime performance, a more upbeat mood, greater health, and an enhanced

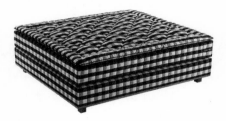

The World's Most Expensive Mattress. The Swedish $59,750 Hastens *Vividus* horsehair, cotton, and wool model. When would you like it delivered?

sense of well-being. Although a week's vacation can deliver that too, its effects won't last as long and it'll cost you lots more.

Willing to give it a try? Want to be wide awake, creative, and dynamic all day long? The only thing you have to do is follow our **Four Essential Keys to Sleeping Well**, which are outlined in this chapter. Tonight, you can begin unlocking the secret to better sleep.

ESSENTIAL KEY #1

> ### Determine your Personal Sleep Quotient (or PSQ) and meet it nightly.

Failing to reach your personal sleep requirement diminishes concentration, productivity, and work quality. If we operated machinery the way we're driving our bodies, we'd be guilty of reckless endangerment. After seventeen to nineteen hours without sleep, your brain activity is similar to someone with a Blood Alcohol Content (BAC) of 0.05 (0.08 being the legal limit for intoxication in most states).

Here's how to determine and meet your "PSQ":

- Pick a bedtime when you're likely to fall asleep quickly that's at least eight hours before you need to get up. Keep to this bedtime for the next week and note when you wake up each morning. You might rise early for a few days if you're used to sleeping less, but that habit will soon give way to longer rest.

- If you need an alarm to wake up, if it's difficult to get out of bed, or if you're tired during the day, eight hours isn't enough sleep for you. Move your bedtime up by fifteen or thirty minutes the next week. Continue doing this each week until you awaken without an alarm and feel alert all day.

> **Imagine what he could do on eight ...**
>
> When asked, "How much sleep do you get?" New York City Mayor Michael Bloomberg responded, "Six hours, if I'm lucky!"

- When you determine what you think is your ideal bedtime, cut fifteen minutes off it to see if you're sleepy the next day. If so, then you've nailed your PSQ. Add those fifteen minutes back, and you're set.

Most adults require between seven and a half and nine hours of sleep to be fully awake and energized all day long. As a rule of thumb, you'll probably have to add one more hour to your current sleep schedule.

Can I sleep too little or too much?

Short-sleepers, people who get six hours or less per night, are more likely to gain weight than those sleeping seven or eight hours, and they are at greater risk for hypertension (heart attacks and strokes), Type II diabetes, cancer, and shortened lifespan. Lack of sleep also has detrimental effects on memory, attention span, energy, and mood.

Studies have shown that sleeping nine hours or more nightly may be associated with as many health problems as short sleep. These conclusions are probably due to underlying illnesses, such as depression, causing people to sleep more, not the other way around.

Can one night of shortened sleep hurt me?

An occasional late night won't cause too much damage, but reducing sleep by just one hour for seven consecutive nights has the same effects as pulling one all-nighter. Sleep debt doesn't dissipate by itself over time, either. Just like credit-card debt, it's cumulative. If you lose several hours of sleep over a few nights, you'll become increasingly more fatigued in the ensuing days even if you resume your normal sleep schedule.

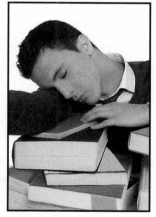

Pulling all-nighters to cram for tests is the students' desperate solution to poor study habits. But lack of sleep foils long-term retention of information and even lowers the body's ability to fight infection. Teachers know to expect lots of coughing and sneezing in class during exam time. Always get a good

A common sight in university lecture halls

night's sleep before any test or interview. According to sleep expert William C. Dement, MD, PhD, if you're in frantic need of more prep time, four hours of sleep is the absolute minimum.

Will my PSQ change over time?

Keep in mind that sleep needs and habits change naturally throughout life. Infants, adolescents, athletes, pregnant women, and senior citizens all have different sleep requirements. In any case, there's no such thing as *too* much sleep. Although you may feel groggy after a long rest because you're waking later when your body temperature is naturally higher, extra shuteye never hurts. (If you have trouble falling asleep or staying asleep, see Chapter 7 for Sure-Fire Strategies to *Sleep for Success!*)

ESSENTIAL KEY #2

> **Go to bed at the same time every night and wake up naturally at the same time every morning, including weekends.**

This means 7 days per week, 365 days per year. Regularity is vital for setting and stabilizing your body's biological clock. It only takes a few weeks to fully synch the hours you spend in bed with the sleepy phase of your clock. When this happens, you won't need an alarm clock to wake you up, and the hours you spend awake will correspond to when you feel most alert and refreshed. In fact, by sticking to a schedule you'll be significantly more alert than if you slept for the same total amount of time at varying hours during the week. And eventually, such regularity will *reduce* the total sleep time required for maximum daytime alertness. Yes, a regular sleep routine will enable you to do just as well on a little less sleep.

British sleep researchers and scientists at Harvard Medical School found that if you alter your sleep schedule by even a few hours, mood deteriorates. Shift-workers in particular may experience more anxiety and depression partly because they're out of synch with their biological clocks.

When should I sleep?

As long as you meet your PSQ without interruption and your boss isn't a stickler for when you show up, it doesn't matter when you bunk down or wake up. Despite what your grandma used to say, sleep prior to midnight isn't better or worth more than sleep after midnight. (She was just trying to get you in before curfew.) Although the first few hours may be more restful in terms of deep (delta) sleep and the secretion of growth hormone, it doesn't matter what time is on the clock when it occurs. Length and regularity of sleep are what count. Of course, it's easier to be sleepy when it's dark and alert when it's light, since sunlight is one of the key determinants of the sleep/wake cycle.

Am I most alert when I first wake up?

Even with adequate rest, don't expect to wake up bright-eyed and bushy-tailed, as the cliché goes. Your body is designed to gradually become more alert, reaching a high point in late morning and again in the late afternoon or early evening. So if you must be at your best first thing in the morning, adjust your schedule accordingly.

For example, morning newscasters should be in bed by 9:00 PM and up by 5:00 AM to be optimally alert for an 8:00 AM camera call. And they should maintain that schedule even when they're off. If they stay up Friday and Saturday nights to socialize and then sleep in the following mornings, they'll have a bad case of Sunday-night insomnia and Monday-morning dark circles. Sorry Regis, Kelly, Diane, and Matt—there's no way around it.

ESSENTIAL KEY #3

Get your required amount of sleep in one continuous block.

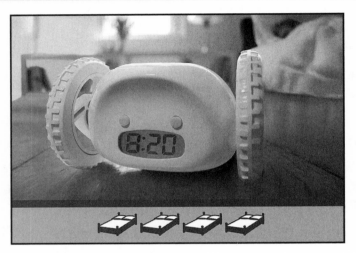

Clocky

This gadget, which will cure your snooze bar addiction, jumps off your nightstand, hides at random, and rings until you find it and shut it off.

Sometimes it's impossible, we know. Any new parent or older guy with prostate woes will tell you so. But so-called "fragmented sleep"—even when endured for hours—is not physically or mentally restorative, and it causes daytime drowsiness. It also dramatically compromises learning, memory, productivity, and creativity. In fact, six hours of continuous sleep are often more restorative than eight hours of fragmented sleep.

Senior citizens anticipating a night of fragmented sleep often go to bed early, hoping to manage eight hours of total sleep within a ten-hour period. But as we've seen, that's a waste of time. So don't let yourself doze on and off for hours. Limiting your time in bed to your PSQ, and not a minute (or twenty) more, will eventually bring greater benefits. Many people use snooze bars thinking that they'll get an extra hour of sleep after the first alarm goes off. Wrong! If you set the alarm to ring every fifteen minutes for an hour, at best, you might get eighteen to twenty minutes worth of fragmented sleep. It's much better to go to bed one hour earlier and wake up naturally.

ESSENTIAL KEY #4

Make up for lost sleep as soon as possible.

As if credit debt wasn't enough, every hour that you're awake you're also building sleep debt. Every two hours of wakefulness require a repayment of one hour of sleep. It's a 2:1 ratio. That's why the general rule is after sixteen hours of being awake you'll need eight hours of sleep. When you violate this rule, sleep debt accumulates very quickly. Before long, you'll crash (hopefully not on the road), you'll get sick, or you'll perform very poorly.

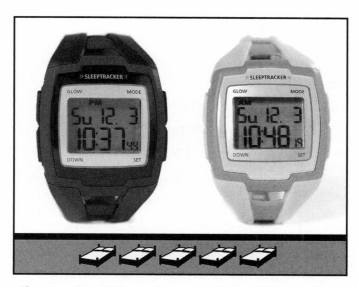

Sleeptracker PRO monitors your body while you sleep. It gently wakes you up when it determines your body is ready. You're left feeling awake, refreshed, and well-rested. Sleeptrackerpro.com

Here's how to make up for lost sleep:

- Don't try to replace it all at once. If you skipped a night, don't try to sleep for fourteen to sixteen hours the next night. That's just about impossible because your long-established biological clock is pre-programmed to put you to sleep and wake you up at a set time every day. Instead, apportion your sleep debt out over the next few days until you feel better.

- Catch up on sleep by going to bed earlier rather than sleeping later. If you sleep later, it will make it harder to get to sleep the following night at the usual hour.

- Don't try to make up for large sleep losses during the week by sleeping in on the weekend. This is like trying to get fit or lose weight by doing all your exercising or dieting on Saturdays and Sundays. Your brain doesn't have a separate biological clock for weekends. Changing your sleep/wake times disturbs your body's natural rhythms. If you sleep until noon on Sunday, for instance, you won't be very tired come your regular bedtime. Maybe you'll doze off sometime after midnight, but just a few short hours later your alarm will jerk you back to consciousness and you'll have to crawl to work with the Monday-morning blahs. You'll have induced jetlag without leaving your zip code.

- Try napping to pay back your sleep debt. However, be careful not to nap too long or too late in the day, or you'll further disturb your sleep cycle. (For more information on finding your "naptitude," see Chapter 8.)

- Whenever your sleep is significantly disturbed, return to your regular schedule as soon as possible. For years of accumulated sleep debt, it may take as long as four to six weeks until you're in the black. But the resulting alertness, mental and physical performance, and enjoyment of life will be more than worth the discipline it took to get there. As you can see, the cure for sleep loss is painless and pleasurable. It just takes a little discipline.

In sum, determine and meet your Personal Sleep Quotient, establish a regular bedtime schedule, get one long block of continuous sleep, and be sure to make up for lost sleep. Now you've got the keys to a brighter, more productive you!

7

Sure-Fire Strategies to Sleep for Success!

We asked sleep-deprived adults why they can't seem to get enough rest at night. Here's a sampling of what they told us:

"I get hungry right before bed and end up eating a big meal."

"My bedroom is hot and stuffy, my mattress sags, and the neighbors are noisy."

"My mind is racing, I'm tense, and I just can't seem to calm myself."

"I've got so much work to do that my bed looks like my desk. In fact, I woke up the other morning with a Post-It note stuck to my chest."

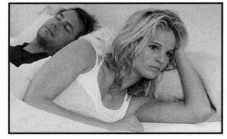

Can't sleep? Maybe it's him. Twenty-three percent of couples sleep apart.

"I'm so frustrated when I wake up at night that I start worrying how I'm going to make it through the next day, and then I can't fall back to sleep."

Do any of these predicaments sound familiar? There are many factors—more than you probably realize—that seriously affect the quantity and quality of our sleep. To hone in on your specific problems, ask yourself these three questions:

- What have I done during the day (e.g., How much caffeine have I had)?

- How's my bedroom environment (e.g., Is it cool enough)?

- How's my attitude (e.g., Am *I* cool enough)?

Fortunately, there are antidotes—proven strategies—that will enable you to overcome common sleep obstacles so you'll be able to *Sleep for Success!* Let's look at some of them within the framework of the three above questions.

THE DAYTIME DO'S FOR NIGHTTIME DOZE

Buzz Off: Avoid caffeine after 2:00 PM

Caffeine stimulates your metabolism, which keeps you awake and alert. It's the magic bullet that allows "sleepy you" and millions of other people to make it through the day. Caffeine is the most widely used drug in the world. Yep, it's a drug (albeit legal) consumed by 85 percent of Americans. Unfortunately, caffeine is a major cause of insomnia, more so than any other food or beverage. The omnipresence of Starbucks and coffee breaks doesn't make it easy, but any coffee (or caffeinated tea, soda, energy drink, or chocolate bar) after 2:00 PM will probably disrupt your sleep. Caffeine has a 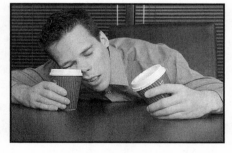 half-life of six hours, which means that six hours after your last sip, half the caffeine is still in your body. If you've had several cups during the day, the effect is cumulative. Consuming more than 300 mg, which is three cups of coffee, cola, or energy drink, will likely affect your sleep. However, it can take *much* less for some individuals—even just one cup of coffee in the morning or a cola at lunch can be disruptive. Everyone's sensitivity to caffeine is different, but it generally increases with age.

> *Limit your caffeine servings to three cups or 300mg daily—all before 2 PM*
>
> *Tips to reduce caffeine intake:*
>
> - Drinking tea? Make one cup with a fresh tea bag, and then throw the tea out. Pour another cup over the same bag for reduced caffeine.
> - Try naturally caffeine-free herbal tea.
> - In the mood for a hot beverage? Have an Ovaltine.

Caffeine not only makes it more difficult to fall asleep, but it also increases the frequency and duration of nighttime awakenings. After a poor night's sleep, you have no choice but to rely on more caffeine to get you through the next day. Then, when it's time to go to bed, your heart is racing, you can't sleep, you wake up exhausted in the morning, and you reach for more caffeine. Sound like a familiar cycle? **Let's break it.**

To gauge the effect caffeine is having on your sleep, eliminate all caffeine from your diet for one week. Although it'll be hard at first, you'll likely find this change allows you to sleep soundly at night and be more productive during the day. If you drink five or more cups daily, you have a dependency problem and will likely find it difficult

> **Good News for Chocoholics: A (small) piece of dark chocolate a day can keep the doctor away.** Dark chocolate can significantly reduce inflammation of the inner lining of the arteries that leads to cardiovascular disease. So, treat yourself to a small piece (0.23 ounces) of dark chocolate. Your sleep will not be affected by that small amount of caffeine.☺

to go cold turkey, so gradually taper off your caffeine consumption. Cut it in half each successive day and substitute a glass of unsweetened fruit juice or water. Women should note that a high intake of caffeine may make it more difficult to become pregnant and can affect the health of the fetus. And if you have any type of heart irregularity, you certainly should be avoiding caffeine, which raises your blood pressure and can induce cardiac arrhythmias. If you miss your cup o' Joe, it's okay to gradually add a small portion of mild or decaf coffee back into your diet. But if you're sleeping well, you'll likely not need any caffeine to make it through the day.

Last Call: *Avoid alcohol three hours before bed*

Many people believe that a nightcap facilitates sleep, but that's a tired old wives' tale. Alcohol is not a sedative—it's a central nervous system suppressant and in quantities becomes a stimulant.

A drink after work or with dinner is fine because your body will have plenty of time to absorb the alcohol. But if you drink within three hours of

> **Cocktail lovers beware!**
> Heavy drinkers have fragmented sleep and are in danger of permanently damaging their pre-programmed sleep system.

bedtime, it will destroy the quality of your rest. Alcohol causes you to wake up in REM sleep every ninety minutes, so throughout the night you'll be continually shaken *and stirred*. And be warned that mixing alcohol with sleeping pills or tranquilizers can be *lethal*.

Butt Out: *Quit smoking for instant rest*

Nicotine is an even stronger stimulant than caffeine. It makes it hard to fall asleep and maintain sleep. The reason nicotine causes you to lie awake at night is that your body is actually experiencing withdrawal symptoms—craving another hit. Smoking also worsens snoring and may cause life-threatening sleep apnea. Aside from its carcinogenic

> **Fill the vacuum:**
> Commit to quitting and fill the void with chewing gum, sipping fruit juice, and exercising.

properties, nicotine increases blood pressure and heart rate and stimulates brain activity. Several studies clearly demonstrate that sleep improves immediately when subjects stop smoking. Two-pack-a-day smokers who quit cut the time they lie awake at night in half.

Eat Well: The skinny on sleep

As a nation, we're fatter, lazier, and sleepier than ever. If you think we're being dramatic, take a look at the fats, er, facts: 63 percent of Americans are overweight, having a body-mass index (BMI) over 25; 31 percent are obese (BMI over 30); and child obesity has more than tripled in the past two decades. Each year about 300,000 Americans die from obesity, making it one of the country's biggest killers. But what does being fat have to do with sleeping? More than you think.

> "The epidemic of obesity is paralleled by a silent epidemic of reduced sleep duration, with shortened sleep linked to increased risk of obesity in adults and in children as young as five."
> —*Francesco Cappuccio, MD*

There's a significant link between sleep deprivation and the risk of obesity. People getting less than four hours of sleep per night are 73 percent more likely to be obese than those getting seven to nine hours. Granted, the correlation goes both ways; people who are obese often have difficulty sleeping due to discomfort and medical problems such as sleep apnea. Nonetheless, there is a strong link between the two. And this is true for children as well as adults.

Staying in bed longer can actually keep you from gaining weight! The less sleep you're getting, the less efficiently this whole appetite-regulation system works. Many people make the mistake of thinking they're hungry when they're actually sleepy. Instead of a snack, they need some shuteye. Once you understand this, you can begin to use sleep to control and even lose weight.

A study at the University of Chicago determined that even among healthy men and women with average BMIs, those who slept less than six hours per night experienced hormonal changes that could affect their future body weight and overall health. These short-sleepers had to produce 30 percent more insulin than normal sleepers just to maintain regular blood-sugar levels. That alone predisposed them to gaining weight. Aside from the chemical changes that occur when you're not sleeping well, there are many emotional and behavioral shifts that also happen, including an erosion of motivation and coordination that, in turn, can make exercising or any physical activity difficult or unappealing.

The skinny on sleep is simple: ignore the common perception that those who sleep for eight hours or more are fat and lazy. Instead, look at it this way: the time you spend in bed is time you won't spend eating. Beyond that, sleeping helps your body better police itself. The best diet may not be Atkins or Jenny Craig; it's getting one additional hour of sleep every night. If you do that and you're currently overweight, expect to lose an average of one pound per week, all else being constant.

Be Active: Exercise between 5:00 and 7:00 PM

Exercise strengthens your heart, lowers blood pressure, and reduces stress. It also raises endorphin levels. Endorphins are natural mood elevators produced by the brain in response to physical activity. They reduce pain, relax muscles, suppress appetite, and produce feelings of overall well-being. Plus, they deepen sleep and make it more efficient and restful.

Ask busy executives to recommend the best time to exercise, and they'll typically respond "early morning." Wrong answer. An extra hour of sleep does more for your health than running around in a half-awake state. Your body temperature is also relatively low in the AM, making it more likely that you'll trip or strain a muscle because you're not fully alert or warmed up. Even when you do

> **Naps Rule**
>
> If you *really* need a nap, keep it short. Fifteen to twenty minutes is max in order to avoid sleep problems at night.

manage to log eight hours of shuteye, you should always loosen up for fifteen to thirty minutes before early-morning exercise in order to dissipate the fluid that accumulates during the night between spinal disks. If you don't ease into the activity, you'll risk lower back pain and even herniating a disk.

The best time to work out is between 5:00 and 7:00 PM. Exercising during these times is more likely to enhance the depth of your nighttime sleep. But avoid strenuous exercise (except pleasurable sex!) within three hours of bedding down. That's because exercise elevates core body temperature for five to six hours. In order to feel drowsy and stimulate the release of melatonin, body temperature needs to be dropping.

It's not surprising that athletes experience more delta-wave (deep), restorative sleep than non-athletes. To approximate that kind of rest, exercise moderately at least five days a week for twenty minutes or more. Any aerobic activity, even fast walking, will not only improve your overall health but also the quality and quantity of your sleep.

Don't Nap Unless You Must

Once you've established good nocturnal habits and you're sleeping long and well, you should stop feeling tired in the afternoon. If you still occasionally do, it's better to resist the urge to nap rather than risk upsetting your new, effective sleep cycle. Likewise, if you're a senior citizen, suffer from insomnia, and/or are struggling to get into a consistent sleep pattern, we recommend pushing through the day without a nap. Your nighttime sleep will be better for it. However, if you're burning the candle at both ends, there's a strong flame of evidence that a twenty-minute afternoon power nap will make you more alert and productive and less anxious about getting to sleep later.

Stay Involved: Busy bees catch more z's

Although it sounds contradictory, boredom can actually cause sleep loss.

We see this frequently among the elderly. Poor sleepers tend to spend more time sitting around and watching TV. Good sleepers spend more time working, socializing, and pursuing hobbies. They are motivated and excited by life's opportunities. So stay mentally active by getting involved in things that interest you and make you think. Do crossword puzzles or Sudoku, take a course online or at a local college, join clubs, volunteer at a hospital, school, church or synagogue, or get a part-time job. In short, live a varied life. This will help you feel good about yourself and make it easier to sleep at night.

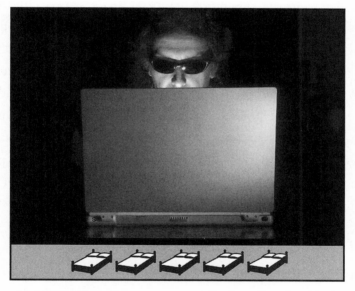

Light-Blocking Glasses are specially formulated to block between 80–98 percent of incident light in the blue range. Blue light makes it difficult for you to fall asleep and is included in daylight spectrum lighting. Electronics like the computer, TV, iPad, etc. emit daylight spectrum lighting. If you must use these products within an hour of bedtime, wear Light-Blocking Glasses to ensure sound slumber.

YOUR BEDROOM ENVIRONMENT

Your bedroom should be a personal sanctuary associated only with rest and relaxation; it shouldn't be a home theater, an auxiliary office, or, even worse, a cafeteria. The quality of your bedroom environment will go a long way in determining the length and quality of your sleep.

Cool Off: Set the thermostat for 65°F

This is the ideal sleeping temperature. If you're used to it being sauna-like, reduce the temperature gradually. A bedroom that's too warm can even induce nightmares as neural activity in the brain will increase in intensity and duration as body temperature rises. Take children, for instance: the tendency is for parents to want to keep them safe and warm. This will result in your kids running into your bedroom in the middle of the night after waking up from a bad dream. Conversely, a room that's too cold keeps your body from fully relaxing because it's trying to protect its core temperature. If 65 degrees feels too frigid, add a blanket, night cap, pair of socks, a special friend, or a warm puppy.

> **Does the humidity matter?**
> Yes! Ideal bedroom humidity is between 60 and 70 percent. Invest in a humidifier, especially in winter months, to make sure your bedroom isn't too dry. A humidifier will also provide a low, constant background hum that neutralizes background noise.

Dim the Lights: Use 45-watt to 60-watt bulbs

Light is one of the most powerful cues for initiating and maintaining wakefulness. The lighting in your bedroom should provide a soft, warm glow. Avoid halogen lamps and fluorescent fixtures. Choose low-wattage, tungsten bulbs (45–60 watts). Also, use a small lamp with a rheostat or dimmer for reading in bed. Gradually lowering the brightness will fatigue your eyes and promote drowsiness.

Once the lights are out, make sure your bedroom is as dark as possible. If city lights are shining through a curtain or shade, try blackout drapes. If light from a bathroom or hall is sneaking under the door, cover the crack with a rolled-up towel. Wearing an eye mask is another alternative. Even the LED digits on your alarm clock have enough luminosity to get through your thin eyelids and disrupt your sleep. If you can dim the display, do so. If not, throw a T-shirt over it. This will also prevent clock watching, which is another sleep disrupter.

Neutralize the Noise: Keep it below 60 decibels

A quiet bedroom is crucial to a good night's rest, but if you live in an urban environment, this can be challenging to accomplish. Even noise as low as 60 decibels, the level of a normal conversation, can stimulate your nervous system. And any sudden or loud sound can put your brain on alert. Most people can adapt to certain recurrent noise like a ticking clock or highway traffic. However, irregular, intermittent sounds like clinking radiators and honking taxis will keep you up. You can mask these disruptive noises with the hum of an air conditioner, humidifier, fan, the static between FM stations, a CD of chirping crickets or rolling surf ... generally any sound that is low and consistent. There are lots of white-noise-generating products on the market, and these solutions are generally less expensive and just as effective.

If you have a partner who snores, try using earplugs or investing in noise-canceling headphones. An occasional poke in the ribs also works, although pinning a sock, with a tennis ball inside, to the back of the nightshirt is more humane. This keeps the perpetrator on his/her side and less likely to snore. Snoring can endanger the heart by narrowing arteries and raising blood pressure. So, if you or your partner snores loudly, consult your physician. The best treatments are usually non-invasive; don't hesitate, you'll live longer!

Decorate Simply: Design a bedroom, not a showroom

Choose muted colors such as neutrals or light pastels for walls and bedding. A light blue ceiling has been found to be soothing. If using brighter accents, avoid contrasting colors because it discourages rest.

> **You're Not the Only One Who Reproduces in Your Bed:** If your old mattress feels heavier when you lift it, it's not your age. The weight of your mattress doubles every ten years due to dust mites!

Keep the bedroom décor to a minimum and reduce visual clutter and stimuli. For example, leave toiletries in the bathroom. Clear off that bureau. Get rid of all those magazines and books on the night table. A plant, a scenic painting, and photos of family are sufficient decorations to balance a bedroom with pleasant memories and produce equally pleasant dreams.

Check Your Undercarriage:
Replace your mattress if it's nearly ten years old

Did you buy your last mattress during the Clinton (or Reagan) administration? Do you wake up stiff or in pain? Are there visible sags and lumps (in the mattress, not you)? Have you recently gotten a better night's sleep somewhere else (maybe even a tent)? If you answered yes to any of these questions, it's probably time for a new mattress. Here are some tips for buying a great one:

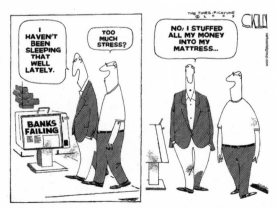

Steve Kelley Editorial Cartoon used with the permission of Steve Kelley and Creators Syndicate. All rights reserved.

- *Try it out*: Don't get bogged down by product claims. Test drive it. When you lie down, your head, neck, and spinal cord should be aligned as if you were standing. Make sure your body is well-supported at all contact points, especially the lumbar region. It doesn't matter if the mattress is classified as soft, medium, or firm as long as it provides a good foundation. If you and your partner prefer different mattresses, consider buying twin beds and pushing them together.

- *Look under the hood*: If you're considering an innerspring mattress, ask about coil count (higher is better). The coils should also be individually pocketed for low motion transfer. Otherwise, you'll be sleeping on a trampoline, and partner movement will disrupt up to 20 percent of your deep sleep. Some foam mattresses generate heat, so ask your mattress dealer if you can test drive one at home for two weeks in the summer to make sure you're comfortable. If you like waterbeds, make sure the vinyl is thick enough to ensure durability and that the bladder has several compartments to reduce seasickness.

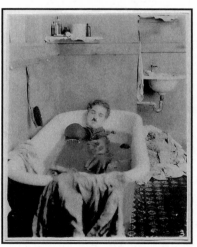

Not the kind of waterbed we're talking about.

- *Give yourself plenty of room:* If you share your bed, be aware that a full-size mattress affords only enough space for a single sleeper who is, at most, 5 feet, 5 inches tall. Thus, you should be considering only queen or king-size models. To be safe, test the mattress with your partner to be sure there's enough room for both of you to sleep comfortably.

- *Spend what it takes:* Buy the best mattress you can afford. A great choice is the Paramount HD (www.paramountsleep. com).

Dress for Rest: Or wear nothing at all

Soft, loose-fitting, breathable garments are ideal. Do not wear nightclothes that are too light or heavy for the season. Avoid fabrics like wool that can irritate your skin. Cotton is a great choice for nightwear because it's comfortable and breathable. Although nightgowns and pajamas are fading out of style, especially among young adults, the more popular sweatpants and sweatshirts can still work as long as they're cottony and comfortable. Be wary, however, of things like hooded sweatshirts because the extra fabric can bunch and disrupt your sleep. When the weather (or the situation) warrants, by all means try sleeping in the nude. It's equally, if not more, conducive to great sleep.

> "I sleep in my wedding ring ..."
> *Kathie Lee Gifford, TV star*

Pick a Perfect Pillow

Just as there are different sleeping styles, there are different pillows to suit them. When selecting a pillow, try it out just like you did your mattress. Make sure it's firm enough to support your head and neck and maintain your spine's normal curve. If you're a folder or stacker, do exactly that in the store. If you usually sleep in a fetal position (most people do), consider a "side-sleeper" pillow. These have two seams so your pillow doesn't come to a point and cause neck discomfort. Although a

> **Do the Pillow Test:** Fold the pillow in half. If it unfolds and returns to its original shape, you have a good pillow. But if your pillow doesn't return to its original shape, throw it out (or put it in the in-law's room☺).

high-quality down or synthetic pillow with high fill power is often preferable, foam, air, water, and buckwheat pillows can provide good support as well.

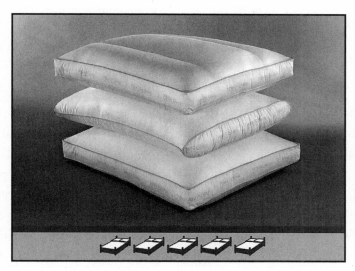

The ***Sleep for Success!***™ pillow collection has breathable fabric with moisture management for an uninterrupted, fully restorative sleep. Its premium-quality natural blend down alternative fill is hypoallergenic. ***Sleep for Success!***™ pillows are available for back, stomach and side sleepers with unique designs for proper neck alignment and a better night's sleep. There is also a **Stress-ease *Comfort Reader Pillow*™** in the collection, as well as a ***Travel Buddy*™** pillow.

Shopping for Super Sheets

Picking a great sheet should start with the feel. Paying too much attention to thread count (the number of threads per square inch of fabric) can steer a consumer into thinking that the higher the thread count, the better quality sheet. Products may be woven with two-ply yarns in order to double the thread count. This allows for the manufacturer to label the product by the total thread count which is actually twice

> For maximum sleep comfort, stick with **100% cotton.** It is an ideal fabric due to its absorbent, breathable quality.

the thread count according to some manufacturers' standards. Although thread count plays a part, the preparation of the yarns (i.e., if the yarns are spun or combed) ultimately determines how the product will feel and wear during its life.

> **Wake Up Fresh**
>
> Air out your bedroom every week to ensure good air quality.
>
> Use dust mite covers (with small pore sizes to block mites) for pillows and mattresses.

Eject the Electronics: Create an information-free zone

This means no computers, TVs, iPads, iPods, or Blackberrys in the bedroom. They create distractions by reminding you of everything else you should be doing and act as secret stressors. However, it's still a good idea to keep a phone by your bed in case of emergency. For some people, installing a home security system helps encourage worry-free sleep.

Read for Pleasure: it will help you calm down and prepare for sleep

To help you wind down, read something for pleasure (that is, not work related). Reading for 30 minutes cuts sleep onset time in half.

Protect Your Privacy: Keep kids out of your bed

If you have young children, don't let them develop the sleep-disrupting habit of crawling into your bed on a regular basis. If they insist, try putting a sleeping bag on the floor. That way, they'll probably return to their own room after a while where the bed is more comfortable.

SAYING SAYONARA TO STRESS

If you've ever tossed and turned in bed festering over your 401K, an unfinished task at work, a "special" co-worker, or an argument you had with a friend or family member, then it shouldn't surprise you to learn that *stress is the number-one cause of insomnia*. In fact, 65 percent of Americans say stress disturbs their sleep. Stressed people have difficulty falling asleep, sleeping deeply, and maintaining sleep throughout the night. They also suffer from early-morning awakenings.

When you feel pressured, your body produces excessive amounts of cortisol, adrenaline, and epinephrine—three of the major stress hormones. The effects of overdosing on these chemicals can be devastating. They can lower your overall immunity and increase your risk of health problems that include high blood pressure, cardiovascular disease, and even cancer. Stress levels are at a record high across the globe. Nevertheless, excessive stress, much like chronic sleepiness, should never be accepted as part of life. If unaddressed, stress and the sleep problems that result will negatively affect your waking hours and may even shorten your life.

Sometimes, sleep helps regulate nervousness and offers an escape from stress, particularly when there's nothing you can do about it. So if you can't cope with it, sleep on it. Here are some short-term solutions for easing stress:

- Take a few deep breaths.
- Take a hike—even if it's just to the water fountain.
- Turn on relaxing music.
- Pet a dog.
- Chew some sugarless gum.
- Eat a small piece of dark chocolate (the chemical phenethylamine elevates mood).
- Count your blessings and focus on the positive things in life.
- Don't sweat the small stuff.
- Call or e-mail a friend with whom you've lost touch.
- Remember a good joke.
- Smile (even if you don't want to) and think a happy thought. Research shows that the physical act of smiling makes people feel happier.
- Think about someone you love.

Take control of your stress! Here are some tips for relaxing in the long term:

- *Meditate:* Many of the brain waves you experience during meditation are the same as those in Stage 2 sleep, so much so that frequent meditators require less nocturnal sleep than non-meditators. Find a quiet space where you won't be disturbed. Sit or lie down. Try repeating a word like "ohm" or "peace." Close your eyes and breathe deeply. As you exhale, silently repeat the word or phrase you've chosen. If you find yourself getting distracted and thinking about a million things, calmly let those thoughts disperse. Don't get agitated if you can't clear your mind. If you find contemplating a word or phrase too difficult, concentrate on your breathing. After ten to twenty minutes, you'll find yourself in a calmer, relaxed state. Just a short period of daily meditation can significantly lower blood pressure. Even mini-meditations throughout the day will help calm you and improve your sleep.

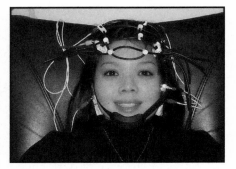

Brain Music Therapy is a highly effective, scientifically based and user friendly technology. It was brought to the US by Galina Mindlin, M.D., Ph.D., Assistant Clinical Professor of Psychiatry, Columbia University, Director BMT Center, NYC. BMT technology starts the brain music therapy program by recording an individual's brain waves. Key rhythms from the recording are translated by a computerized mathematical formula into musical sounds. The results are often compared to classical music, but each is individualized.

- *Visualize:* Imagine a serene place, such as a beach, and actually try to smell the air, touch the sand, and feel the warm sun on your face. Infuse your visualization with positive statements such as "I'm at peace" or "I feel calm."

- *Massage:* Ask a friend or a family member to give you a massage, or make an appointment with a professional therapist. Massage improves circulation and relaxes tense muscles. If you're really cramped for time (pun intended), try Progressive Muscle Relaxation (PMR). Lie down or sit in a quiet, comfortable place. Tense and relax your muscles in groups, starting from the toes and slowly working up to the eye muscles and forehead. Squeeze tightly for five to ten seconds, then release and relax for fifteen to twenty seconds before moving on to the next body part.

- *Aromatherapy:* Hippocrates used aromatherapy to help cure Rome of the plague. If it relaxes you, why not try adding soothing lavender or sage to a hot bath? If you don't have time for a bath, rub some oils on your hands and temples. Another great prop is a lavender eye pillow, which will soothe eyes and temples.

- *Breathe:* Deep breathing is one of the easiest ways to adjust your attitude and the way you're feeling physically. Most people don't breathe properly, even when they're not stressed. If you become overwhelmed at any point during the day, take a quick two-minute breather—literally. Inhale through your nose and then exhale through your mouth making sure that you completely empty your lungs of air. Then breathe in again (deeper this time), exhale (longer this time), and repeat for as long as desired. You'll soon find yourself in a peaceful and composed state of mind.

- *Talk to someone:* Sometimes a brief chat with a friend or coworker, or just a five-minute venting session with a spouse, is all it takes to make you feel better. No humans available? Your pet is nonjudgmental.

- *Exercise:* Any type of physical activity is a great way to alleviate stress. Classes such as step aerobics or kickboxing offer great escapes. They get your heart pumping, raise endorphin levels, and eventually brighten your mood while reducing stress. But even just a walk or an evening bike ride will help clear your mind. Think of it as active meditation.

A pre-sleep routine is key to a good night's sleep.

In order to sleep soundly through the night, your body needs to prepare itself for the long period of inactivity ahead. It needs a buffer between the day's stress and the night's rest. You need to find peace and calm in the hour before bed. Slipping between the sheets and closing your eyes should be the very last part of that ritual. Here's how to ease out of the day:

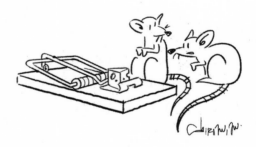

"No thanks. I read somewhere that late night snacking can be bad for your health."

www.CartoonStock.com

Snack Smart: Eat a small, high-carb, low-protein food

If you're hungry, nibble on something high in carbohydrates but low in protein. These types of foods contain glucose, which speeds the amino acid tryptophan to the brain, where it is converted to serotonin, a sleep-inducing neurotransmitter. This process takes forty-five to sixty minutes once the food is eaten. Stay away from anything that causes heartburn or indigestion. Warm milk, being high in protein, is the one exception.

Best/Worst Bedtime Snacks

EAT:	AVOID:
✓ Fiber and whole grains	✓ Alcohol
✓ Crackers	✓ Caffeine (chocolate)
✓ Sparkling water	✓ Spicy food
✓ 2 tbsp hummus with vegetables	✓ Dairy products (cheese, yogurt)
✓ Banana, apple	✓ Meats high in protein (sausage)
✓ Dried fruit and nuts	✓ Processed food or MSG
✓ Peanut butter, almond butter	✓ Garlic
✓ Cereals, oats	

Wash Away the Day: Take a hot (100°F) bath or shower

Just before bed, a warm, soaking shower or a relaxing Jacuzzi will redirect blood from your brain to your skin. This will raise your temperature and make you feel relaxed. Then, when you enter the bedroom (which should be kept at 65°F), your body temperature will plummet. This helps initiate deep sleep.

Slow Down the Brain: Do something mindless

Your brain doesn't have an on/off switch. If you're doing stimulating work until 11:00 PM, don't expect to fall asleep at 11:15. You must give yourself time to wind down. During the thirty to sixty minutes before bed, work on a mindless hobby, read a novel, do light housework like folding laundry, or handwrite a few thank-you notes to people you appreciate.

Forget Your Worries: Accentuate the positive

> **Send Your Worries On A Cruise:** If your mind is buzzing with worries, mentally wrap each one in a package, imagine yourself wading into a stream, and then let each worry package float away.

If you're festering about an upcoming exam, interview or appointment, visualize success. Tell yourself that no matter how worried you are or how much you have scheduled, there's nothing you can do about it until tomorrow.

Stretch for Sleep: Three exercises that promote relaxation

Light exercises, deep breathing, and some yoga poses can help your mind relax, let go of worry, and slip into a deep slumber.

- *Child's pose*: Sit on your calves, rear end on your heels, with the tops of the feet on the floor. Slowly bring your head forward to the ground and place your hands, palms up, alongside your hips. Your neck should be elongated and your abs engaged. Breathe deeply and feel your worries slip away.

- *Table pose*: Get down on your knees and support yourself with your hands so that you resemble a table. Make sure your palms are directly below your shoulders. Your knees should be hip-width apart and toes pointed. Spread your fingers wide for support. Keep your neck extended and fix your gaze several feet in front of you. Hold this pose for fifteen seconds. Focus on your breathing and the opening between your shoulder blades. Now alternate between arching your back like an angry cat and pushing your belly down to the ground. You can also alternate extending your right arm and left leg and vice versa.

- *Corpse pose*: Lie on the floor on your back with feet outstretched in front of you. Heels should be a centimeter apart and feet should fall naturally. Rest your hands comfortably, palms up, beside you. Close your eyes and focus on deep breathing.

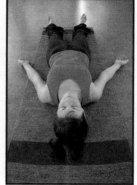

Seven Sleep Worries Put to Rest:

1. What if I don't fall asleep as soon as my head hits the pillow?

It takes a well-rested person fifteen to twenty minutes to fall asleep. If you fall asleep instantly, that's a sure sign you're sleep-deprived.

> "I'm asleep the second my head hits the pillow."
> —*Michael Bloomberg, Mayor, New York City*

2. What if I can't stop tossing and turning?

If you toss and turn, get out of bed! The more time you spend thrashing about, the less quality sleep you'll get. Plus, it may lead you to associate the bedroom with feelings of frustration, discomfort, and unhappiness. Whenever restlessness persists for more than fifteen minutes, go to another room. Walk around, tidy up, star gaze out a window ... basically do anything that is relaxing, moderately boring, or doesn't require concentration. Usually it will take fifteen to twenty minutes for your body to feel sleepy again, at which point you can return to the bedroom.

> **Try hard and you won't succeed...**
> Volunteers who were promised $25 if they could fall asleep quickly took twice as long to nod off as those who weren't paid anything.

3. What if I wake up in the middle of the night and can't get back to sleep?
It's normal to awaken one or two times per night for various reasons. If you're unable to fall back to sleep within fifteen to twenty minutes, then follow the advice above. You'll generally find that you'll get back to sleep sooner than if you had stayed in bed.

4. Am I spending too much time in bed?
Stress, depression, boredom, and even pressure from a partner (e.g., who works a different shift) can all get you into bed earlier and/or out later than you should. Listen to your body and only go to bed when you're tired. Older people, fearing a night of several awakenings and light sleep, often go to bed too early. This only compounds the problem of fragmented sleep. Only stay in bed for as long as you need to feel refreshed. Spending too much time there promotes shallow and disturbed overall sleep.

5. What if I like to fall asleep watching TV?
No matter how pleasurable you may find this, it's usually a bad idea. TV is very engaging and stimulating (with the noteworthy exception of C-Span). In fact, we recommend there not be a TV in your bedroom at all. And, if possible, limit your TV-viewing time during the day as well. Although you may be able to fall asleep with Letterman on, it will likely result in early-morning awakenings during lighter sleep cycles. If you must watch TV, at least set a timer so it's not on all night. (The noise will pull you awake as your sleep gets lighter toward morning.)

6. What if I'm sharing a bed with someone else?
In yet another testament to the profound differences between the sexes, research shows that women sleep less soundly when they share a bed with a romantic partner while men actually sleep better. Perhaps this is why an estimated 23 percent of American couples sleep apart. Women

may have a tougher time sharing a bed simply because men are more likely to snore, or there may be actual brain-wiring differences stemming from a woman's instinctive role as infant caregiver. Most often, it's the woman who gives in and moves to a different bed or room.

When sleeping with someone, we actually condition ourselves to not move as much as if we were in bed alone, which also contributes to fewer restful nights. Keep in mind, however, that if you have a sleeping partner, you're fortunate enough to have your own private sleep doctor who can monitor your breathing. Sexual activity (either making love or masturbation) promotes peaceful, deep sleep.

7. What about letting the family pet into my bed?
Sixty-seven percent of people regularly sleep with their cats and dogs. Fifty-one percent say their sleep is disturbed by their partner, while just 38 percent claim their pets wake them up.

> Has something come between you? 67 percent of couples sleep with a pet.

By the way, women are more inclined to prefer pets in their bed to men, with 55 percent saying their guy is more of a bed hog than their dog or cat. Nonetheless, it's better to give Brutus (the dog!) his own bed on the floor.

8 What's your Naptitude?

Do you get sleepy after lunch? Do your eyelids feel like mini-dumbbells halfway through the afternoon? If so, a nap is an easy, healthful way to quickly boost alertness, concentration, productivity, creativity, and mood. Although napping has acquired a stigma of laziness, even Fortune

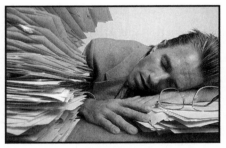

The Boss Is Out: Our bodies are naturally programmed for an afternoon shutdown, regardless of location.

500 companies are waking up to the stress-reducing, efficiency-enhancing importance of this biological process.

According to a Pew Research Center Social & Demographic Trends 2009 survey, thirty percent of adults admit that on any typical day they take a nap. The survey also asked respondents if they had trouble sleeping in the past twenty-four hours—and, not surprisingly, it finds a correlation between nap-taking and trouble sleeping.

So stop being a napaphobe and start working through your inbox after a midday snooze, whistling and looking like you're riding a double-espresso high. Here's how.

WHAT YOU SHOULD KNOW

Napping is not just for newborns and nanas. A British study found that simply anticipating a nap is enough to lower blood pressure. Research in Greece showed that napping lowers the risk of heart attack and stroke, while other studies have yielded similar findings for obesity and diabetes. Napping benefits the mind, too—enhancing creative thinking, boosting cognitive processing, improving memory recall, and generally clearing the cobwebs.

Is a nap right for me?

If you're one of the lucky few who gets adequate sleep every night, you may not need (or be able) to nap. However, for the rest of us, life happens. When sleep is curtailed at night, a nap can be a stop-gap measure to get through the day. Naps can also be part of a well-rested person's normal routine, serving as a natural, midday pick-me-up.

Top 5 Things to Say if You Get Caught Sleeping at your Desk

5. "They told me at the blood bank this might happen."
4. "This is just a fifteen-minute power nap like they raved about in the last time-management course you sent me to."
3. "I wasn't sleeping! I was meditating on the mission statement and envisioning a new paradigm!"
2. "Darn! Why did you interrupt me? I had almost figured out a solution to our biggest problem."
1. "Amen."

Our bodies are programmed with a biphasic sleep pattern, which means they cycle through two periods of drowsiness every twenty-four hours. One is between 2:00 and 4:00 PM, and the other is in the late evening before bed.

The corporate world's answer to the mid-afternoon energy dip has traditionally been a coffee or cola break. However, these caffeinated quick fixes often interfere with the nighttime sleep cycle. A better remedy, when possible, is a short nap.

In Greece, southern Italy, and throughout Latin America, the *siesta* is used to counteract this dip and escape the hottest part of the day. But even in Spain, only 7 percent of the population naps presently. Unlike every other mammal on the planet, we increasingly fight the urge because we're too busy, too stubborn, or too ashamed to admit that we need a rest. But it's time we tuck that thinking away.

How long should I nap?

In theory, you have two options. Depending on how much time you have, a nap of twenty or ninety minutes will leave you refreshed. Why these specific times? While sleeping, your body progresses through five distinct sleep cycles ranging from light (Stages 1 and 2) through delta or slow-wave sleep (Stages 3 and 4) to REM, the deepest of all (Stage 5). A successful nap is one that either takes you through just the first two stages (generally twenty minutes) or one that goes through one complete sleep cycle and awakens you during Stage 2 of the next cycle (usually about ninety minutes). The key is to wake up during a lighter sleep stage in order to feel rejuvenated. Otherwise, you'll feel groggy and more tired and ornery than before. (Note: everybody's individual sleep clock is different, so experiment to find the perfect nap times for you.)

New finding:
Naps can help do the following:

- Speed up the rate at which we learn new information
- Solidify information into long-term memory
- Avoid new information from getting confounded with old information
- Increase motor skill performance by 16 percent if you are sleep- deprived and your nap is long enough to include some REM sleep.

Even a few minutes of napping can be beneficial.

Most napaphobes assume there's no way they can relax, doze off, and get any amount of worthwhile sleep in just twenty minutes. But remember that a nap is *not* the same type of sleep experience you get at night. It's something different, and it must be approached as such.

Think of it this way: Your body is hungry for sleep, but you can't give it a full-course meal during the day. You can, however, serve up a pretty tasty

> **Kids napping is okay.** *Studies show kids who nap during the day are less likely to put up a fight at bedtime.*

snack—one that replenishes its energy store, takes the edge off its appetite, and allows it to continue functioning without distraction. Viewed this way, it's easier to see how even a twenty-minute nap can satisfy the body.

Won't napping make it harder for me to fall asleep at night?

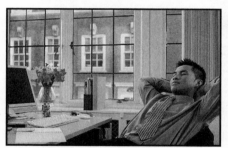

Just closing your eyes for twenty minutes can be restorative.

Only if you break the rules we just outlined and wake up four hours later in a pool of drool. Be careful, however, if you have a history of insomnia. If so, napping may not be a good idea. Experiment with a twenty-minute nap first to see if it has any effect. Some insomniacs actually find that napping reduces their sleep anxiety and allows them to doze off more easily at night. Incidentally, people who skip naps don't sleep any better or longer at night than those who do nap.

Does napping help make up for lost sleep?

Yes, but it should be considered an alternative—not an antidote—for bad sleep habits. While it's nourishing and even luxurious to nap, and we should all try to do so as often as possible, there are many times when we can't turn off the world for even twenty minutes. That's why consistent, restful, nighttime sleep is so important and why you should continue to make that your priority. Even perfect sleepers (both of you out there raise your hands!) can continue to use napping as a tool to maximize performance.

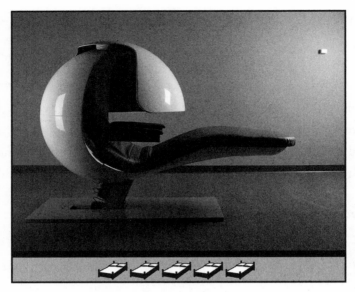

Nap to the future: "The Energy Pod"

Grabbing some Zs on your lunch break could be easier than you think: tell your boss you have "an appointment" and go enjoy a blissful twenty minutes of shuteye. More and more spas (many in corporate buildings) are investing in state-of-the-art napping equipment in an effort to cater to the overtired working world. Those like Rejuvenate Salon in Atlanta offer everything from a twenty-minute power nap in a reclining chair "that feels like zero gravity" to a nap of any length in the Alpha 2010, a pod that offers a "complete spa-napping experience." We're talking dry heat on your body, a cool breeze on your face, aromatherapy oils (you can choose your favorite), meditative sounds, scented eye pillows, and a private curtained room ... all for only $14.

"Sorry, I tried, but I just can't nap ..."

Nobel Prize winners, presidents, distinguished scientists, and athletes all nap: Albert Einstein, John Kennedy, Winston Churchill, Thomas Edison, Lance Armstrong—there's no reason you can't, too. If you're having trouble napping, you might be too caffeinated, there may be too much light (or noise) in the room, or you may harbor subconscious fears of getting caught. (Or, more positively, you may be sufficiently rested and not need a nap.)

Close the door, turn down the lights, and put in some earplugs. If you don't have the luxury of privacy, consider a bathroom stall, your car, a corporate nap room (if you're so lucky), or a bench in a nearby park. (Whenever you nap, you should set a small alarm in order to wake up at the prescribed time.)

Most important, try to forget about the to-do list in your head. Write everything down if it'll help clear it, and tell yourself that although you may feel overwhelmed now, when you wake up you'll be better prepared to start crossing things off.

What if I'm sleepy after napping?

If you just take a twenty-minute power nap, there is no risk of grogginess because you will not enter the deeper stages of sleep. However, after a long nap you may feel groggy due to waking up during a deep sleep cycle.

What ingredients are necessary for a perfect nap?

Time: If you don't make time to nap, you won't have time to nap. Don't blame your lifestyle, job, or the number of hours in the day. If you have time to run to Starbucks for a latte, you have time to nap. Just as with anything else, it's a matter of prioritizing.

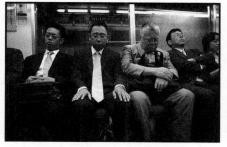

Subway Sleepers: Commuters in Japan

Clear Mind: Sweep your head of "nap blockers." Put your cell phone on silent, set an alarm that you can trust, and put your computer into sleep mode. If you have to, make a list of things you need to handle as soon as you wake up. Then close your eyes and drift off.

Darkness: Do everything you can to block the light in your napping place, even if it means using an eye mask.

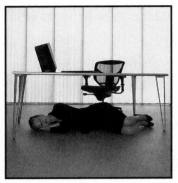

Feel free to sleep around at the office.

Quiet: Noise, unless it's white noise, will ruin your chances of taking a quality nap. Use earplugs or noise-canceling headphones; turn on a fan, an air conditioner, or something else that generates ambient noise.

Comfort: You may not be able to get into your PJs and hop into bed, but get as close (and as comfortable) to that scenario as you can. Lie down. Otherwise, use a mat or just sit back in your chair. Support your head and limbs so you won't jerk yourself awake once you get past Stage 1 sleep (which lasts two to five minutes). Your body associates certain positions with sleep, so anything you can do to trick it into thinking it's bedtime will help.

Cool: Sleep researchers recommend a chilly 65–68 degrees Fahrenheit for optimal nighttime sleeping. This is because good nocturnal sleep is triggered by low body temperature. Naps, however, usually occur at a time of the day when our core body temperature is at its highest, so try to cool down a bit. You should be comfortable—not too hot or cold.

Guiltlessness: Feel safe. Feel peaceful. Feel entitled to take this small amount of time for yourself.

Napping keeps you calm. Matt Walker of the Sleep and Neuroimaging Laboratory at the University of California at Berkeley showed test subjects the faces of people expressing anger, fear, and happiness. They showed the faces at noon and at 6 pm. They found that subjects were significantly more upset by angry and fearful faces later in the day, *unless* they'd had a ninety-minute lunchtime nap in which they experienced REM sleep.

PART Four

New Research that Provides Helpful Solutions to Common Sleep Challenges

9
Sleep from Birth through Childhood

You're a parent, and you're tired—very tired. You want what's best for your child, but you also want what's best for you. So how can you ensure that everyone gets the sleep they need and stays safe and healthy? This chapter provides the tools, tips, and information to help you achieve that. It's a primer for how parents and children of any age can get more healthful rest. But remember: while this advice is supported by studies, popular literature, and professionals, every child and family is unique, and deviations from "average" should be expected. So read on, use what makes sense, and have your entire family getting *Sleep for Success!*

How can I tell if my child is getting enough sleep?

For the first three to four months of life, assume that your baby is sleeping adequately. At this age, sleep is biologically rather than environmentally driven; a baby doesn't care if it's dark or light, if everyone else is sleeping or awake, or whether the clock says 2:00 PM or 4:00 AM. He sleeps and wakes when he needs to—not unlike your Great Uncle Chester.

Newborns have so much to learn they do it in their sleep: Dr. William Fifer, Columbia University, found that newborns can be classically conditioned in their sleep! A tone was played and followed by a puff of air into the sleeping newborn's faces, causing the babies to squeeze their eyelids. Eventually, the tone alone evoked the blinking response. This type of training might someday be used to test for developmental conditions.

After the first few months, environmental and parental cues begin having more influence. At this stage, the most important thing is to keep a *consistent* sleep schedule. Although bedtimes will naturally vary a bit, daytime naps and overall night sleep should be kept fairly regular.

To help you develop a consistent sleep schedule for your child, here are some general, age-group patterns and a few helpful tips:

Age Group	Total Sleep Need	Sleep at Night	Sleep During Day
Newborns *1–2 months*	15–18 hours	2–3 hours at a time, any time of day	
Infants *3–11 months*	14–15 hours	9–12 hours	1–4 naps, from 30 minutes to 2 hours
Toddlers *1–3 years*	12–14 hours	10–14 hours	0–1 naps
Preschoolers *3–5 years*	11–13 hours	9–13 hours	0–1 naps
Children *5–12 years*	10–11 hours	10–11 hours	Usually none
Teens *13–17 years*	8.5–9.25 hours	8.5–9.25 hours	Usually none

Don't wait until your child is tired to put him to bed. Have you ever seen a mother playing with her child and as he begins to fuss she declares him "tired" and announces it's "time for bed?" Actually, the time to tuck him in is *before* this happens. For a baby, that's usually after about two hours of wakefulness; for a four to eight-month-old, after about three hours. This means you should start soothing and quieting the child after one to two hours of wakefulness.

Naptime No-No's
Common mistakes parents make

Delaying sleep
Four-month-olds should go to sleep after about 2 hours of
wakefulness, and 8-month-olds after about 3 hours.

Motion sleeping
Car rides, strollers, and swings are helpful on occasion for
encouraging sleep, but once the child nods off, take her home
or turn off the swing for some good, motionless sleep.

Inconsistent soothing
Do you rock your newborn to sleep before putting
her down, or do you give her a hug and set her in her
crib awake? Whatever you do, be consistent.

Too-short naps
Sleep restores the body and the mind. Naps less than 30
minutes don't allow your child to experience all the different
stages and benefits of sleep that help with restoration.

From *Healthy Sleep Habits, Happy Child* by Marc Weissbluth, M.D.

Don't deprive your child of naps. This is one of the most notable causes of overtired children, especially when they're old enough for parents to start them in organized afternoon activities. Children will not make up for this lost nap time by sleeping longer at night and are likely to become overtired and fussy. If your child *does* miss a nap, however, it's better to forget about it than try to make it up later in the day. Doing that will throw off the nighttime sleep schedule.

Remember that when they're wired, they may be tired. A hyper-aroused child may actually be an overtired child. Often when kids are low on sleep, their

When to Worry

Normal breathing in an infant consists of 20 to 60 breaths per minute and can include pauses of up to 10 seconds. This can be frightening for new parents, but it's nothing to worry about. If, however, your child's breathing pauses (nighttime or daytime) are longer than 10 seconds or if he begins to change color (a blue tint indicates lack of oxygen), call 911 immediately.

body responds by producing such hormones as adrenaline and cortisol. This causes them to appear energized when they're really exhausted.

Be aware that an earlier bedtime can mean more sleep. If you put your child to bed earlier, you would expect him to wake earlier, right? Wrong. Research shows that tucking a child in sooner actually causes them to sleep later. An early bedtime (6:00 to 8:00 PM for those over four months) is an easy way to ensure sufficient sleep.

Never wake a sleeping baby. This will disturb his sleep continuity, an important part of emotional, psychological, and physical development. Infants will wake on their own, usually when they need to be fed (again, just like your Great Uncle Chester). The only exception to the no-waking rule is if your child is over four months of age and you're trying to develop a regular, age-appropriate sleep pattern.

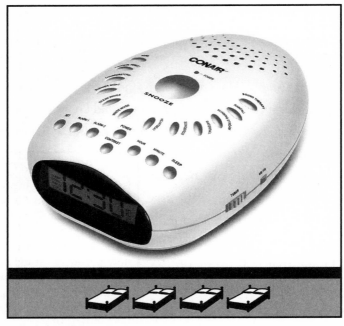

Conair Infant Sound Machine offers 10 soothing sounds from flowing streams to tropical birds, specially designed to lull your baby to sleep.

What disrupts a child's sleep most?

Obstructive Sleep Apnea: At three to four years of age, children are at highest risk for Obstructive Sleep Apnea. OSA affects about 1 percent to 3 percent of children and involves abnormal nighttime breathing due to a partially blocked airway. Some things that accompany OSA include snoring, breathing pauses, enlarged tonsils and adenoids, asthma, allergies, obesity, mouth-breathing, and excessive daytime sleepiness. If you think your child has OSA, call your pediatrician.

Parasomnias: In the early school-age years, as REM sleep becomes less common and Sleep Stages 3 and 4 lengthen, it's not unusual for kids to develop parasomnias. These include sleepwalking, sleep-talking, bedwetting, and night terrors. They usually occur within the first few hours of sleep and specifically during, or as an arousal from, Stage 4 sleep. They last a few minutes to an hour and often end with the

> *Terrorized by Night Terrors*
>
> "Taylor had night terrors when she was 3 to 4 years old. She would wake up screaming like she was having a bad dream. One time she actually had a seizure, and we ended up in the emergency room. She had a brain scan, and it was a scary time. But the doctors couldn't find any reason for it happening. I slept with her pretty much every night after that to calm her in case it happened again, but she eventually outgrew them."
> —*Sandy V., Renton, Washington*

child falling back to sleep peacefully. Parasomnias generally fade by adolescence but can reappear with sleep-deprivation. With the exception of bedwetting, it's best not to wake the child from a parasomnia or to mention it to them later. This will add to their distress and promote negative feelings about bedtime. Here's a bit more information about each of these parasomnias:

Sleep-talking is very common, occurring in about half of children age three to ten at least once per year. It's not harmful to the child, and it's nothing to worry about (unless he's reciting mathematical equations, at which time you should start thinking MIT).

Sleepwalking is also fairly common, occurring in 5 percent to 15 percent of kids ages six to sixteen at least once or twice per year. Parents of sleepwalkers should make sure the house is safe at night—nothing to trip on or fall from, locked doors, latched windows, and no sharp objects. Although waking a sleepwalker is not dangerous per se, waking a sleepwalking child will usually add to their confusion and distress and make it likely to happen again. Doing so may also cause your child to become self-conscious and dread bedtime. The best solution is to gently lead her back to bed.

Bedwetting occurs in 20 percent of children at age four, 10 percent at age five, and 5 percent at age ten. Its cause is unknown, but it's more common in boys than girls. It also seems to be hereditary and often accompanies late bedtimes and severe allergies or breathing problems. If your child frequently wets the bed, talk to him about it, emphasizing that it's not his fault. (Make sure no one in the family teases him.) Keep him from drinking too much in the evening and be sure he goes to the bathroom before bed. Use positive reinforcement such as a sticker chart for dry nights. If his bedwetting persists after age six, consult your pediatrician.

Night terrors are not the same as nightmares. Night terrors occur during Stage 4 sleep (rather than REM), and the child usually has no recollection of them the next day. They are a spontaneous activation of the child's amygdala (the fear center of the brain) and cause your child to experience the feeling of fear without having an actual nightmare. During an episode, she may scream, kick, and appear very distressed, but night terrors are not harmful, and the child will usually grow out of them. Just make sure she's safe—nothing to bang or hit nearby that could hurt her—and be as comforting as you can.

Another common sleep-disrupter among youngsters is Restless Legs Syndrome (RLS). This is a tingly or crawling sensation in the legs that prompts them to move or flex their limbs to relieve the feeling. Children may describe it as "itchy bones" or "creepy crawly." RLS is more common in those with iron-deficient anemia and can often be relieved with exercise, dietary measures, and sometimes medication.

A similar condition is called Periodic Limb Movement Disorder (PLMD). Sufferers briefly awaken at night after repeatedly moving their limbs to soothe tingling sensations. If your child complains of these feelings and appears sleepy during the day, have him avoid caffeinated beverages, encourage him to exercise, and make sure he's eating a healthful diet that includes sufficient amounts of iron.

Yet another disrupter of sleep is Attention Deficit Hyperactive Disorder (ADHD). It affects 5 percent to 10 percent of children in the United States. Symptoms include difficulty concentrating for any length of time and completing schoolwork. ADHD typically develops before age seven and has nothing to do with how a child is raised; it's simply related to chemicals and wiring in the brain. Although many parents of ADHD children claim their kids sleep less and take longer to doze off than others, studies show this is not the case. They may, however, wake up more frequently during the night, although this could be a side effect of their medication and should be discussed with your pediatrician. Also, be aware that the sleep/ADHD connection works both ways: not only can ADHD cause more frequent night-wakings, but sleep problems can exacerbate ADHD. So either way, take all the necessary steps to make sure your son or daughter is getting sufficient sleep.

It should be noted that many kids who can't stay focused in school are mistakenly identified by teachers as having ADHD, when the real problem is lack of proper sleep.

How early should I start a child on a regular schedule?

Jodi Mindell and her colleagues at Saint Joseph's University and The Children's Hospital of Philadelphia, Pennsylvania, found that a regular bedtime routine resulted in significant reductions in problematic sleep behaviors for infants and toddlers. There were significant improvements in time-to-sleep onset and night awakenings. Sleep continually increased, and mommies were even in a better mood. All the mothers did was institute a nightly three-step bedroom routine for two weeks. This included a bath, massage, and quiet activities (cuddling, singing lullabies) then lights out after thirty minutes. Take a hint, Mom and Dad, from these results. Be regular and *you'll* sleep like a baby.

What are the biggest myths about children and sleep?

Teething disturbs it: Researchers have yet to find any direct link between teething and the sleep-disrupting symptoms that parents attribute to it. One possible explanation: a child's teeth generally appear between five and ten months, which is the same time that waking and fearfulness due to separation anxiety (a normal developmental stage) begins.

Growing pains can disrupt sleep: According to the American Academy of Pediatrics, "even at the peak of the adolescent growth spurt, a youngster's rate of growth is too gradual to be painful." So what are these nighttime "pains" that youngsters complain about? Probably just soreness from exercise and excessive playfulness during the day.

Snoring means they're sleeping deeply: Healthful sleep in children and adults should *not* be accompanied by snoring. In fact, one study associated snoring with daytime drowsiness, bedwetting, decreased school performance, morning headaches, mood and personality changes, and weight problems. If you're worried about your child's snoring, ensure that he or she is getting enough sleep, refer to the symptoms described earlier in this chapter for OSA, and consult your pediatrician.

> **Why Doesn't My Preemie Match These Sleep Patterns?**
>
> If your baby was born prematurely, expect normal sleep patterns and behavioral developments to occur according to his *due date* rather than his *birth date*. For example, preemies tend to regularize their night-sleep about six weeks after their due date, while full-term babies develop it six weeks after their birth date. Our sincere best wishes to those parents enduring this!

Switching to solid food helps babies sleep through the night: Studies comparing breastfed, bottle-fed, solid-fed, and even IV-fed children have shown that sleep remains fairly constant. (There is one exception, though: breastfed babies tend to wake more frequently for feedings than bottle-fed infants.)

Can a child's sleep problems be the parents' fault?

Yes. As with everything else in life, your child learns from you. Although she instinctively knows how to sleep, she will acquire her sleep habits from you. So one of the best things you can do to help her sleep better is to prioritize and regularize your sleep, too.

What is the most important thing to remember about kids and sleep?

Consistency. As soon as your child is about three to four months old, it's vital to develop an age-appropriate sleep schedule and to *stick to it!* Children

> "Sleep problems in children are both preventable and treatable."
> —*J.A. Owens and J. Mindell*

with consistent schedules are more well-rested and easier to manage at bedtime because their body is trained to sleep and wake at certain times.

You should also devise a bedtime routine that's about thirty minutes long and includes soothing activities such as taking a bath and reading. These activities will help calm your child down and relax his nervous system, as opposed to activities like watching TV that stimulate them and keep them tossing and turning at night.

New moms should forget about getting adequate sleep, right?

When a child is younger than six weeks, it's very hard to get good, continuous rest. Although the first few days at home are deceiving, with baby sleeping sixteen to eighteen hours per day in four to five-hour increments, things quickly change. For most of those six weeks, the child's longest sleep period will only be two to three hours and can occur at any time. Here are the keys to a well-rested mommy:

Double Trouble

"During the first 4 months after my twins were born, I got only 4 hours of sleep nightly. I tried napping when they napped, but I was a mess ... feeling like a zombie and forgetting to buckle the girls into their car seats, almost running over the stroller while backing up the truck (multiple times!), picking up the child I had just nursed and trying to nurse her again (hmmm, I wonder why she isn't hungry?), falling asleep during breastfeeding, etc. Cognitive reasoning went out the window."
—*Deanne D., Bellevue, WA*

Twins tip: Try to get both children on identical sleep schedules as soon as possible.

Nap whenever possible. As tempting as it may be to do chores and run errands while baby naps, resist the urge. To be a good parent you need to be a well-rested parent. So nap when baby naps. Ideally, household duties can be accomplished while the baby is awake with the help of your spouse, relatives, babysitters, or, in the case of multiple births, the National Guard.

Stay with breast milk. It's always tempting for nursing moms to switch to formula as their sleep-deprivation builds. But the American Academy of Pediatrics recommends that mothers breastfeed exclusively for the first six months and, in fact, suggest continuing for twelve months or longer if possible.

Use the "On 3/Off 3" system. To minimize sleepless nights, try alternating the parent in charge. In other words, put Mom on duty for three nights, put Dad on watch for the next three, and so on. For Mom's nights off, prepare expressed breast-milk bottles in advance. And for either parent's nights off, make sure to fully separate yourself from the child. In other words, trust your partner to care for the baby, even going as far as to sleep in a different part of the house where you won't hear him crying (the baby, that is, not your spouse). Don't think this is selfish. By ensuring that you're well rested and healthy, you're being the best caregiver you can be. If Dad claims he might not hear the baby crying, tell him that might be a myth. Most men's parental radar is just as sensitive as a woman's. This system can also work for separated couples (early in life, babies can sleep anywhere), or for single moms or dads with a willing relative or assistant.

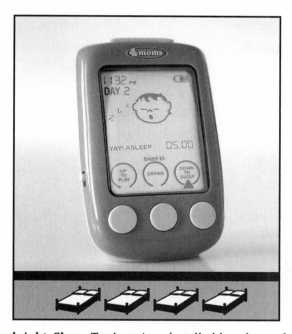

Goodnight Sleep Trainer is a handheld gadget which contains a progressive timer to help parents know how long to wait before comforting baby. The device is accompanied by a website to track sleep progress. This product relieves parents of some worries about how their child is sleeping.

Be patient, the end is near. After six weeks, your child's circadian rhythm will begin to mature, and her night sleep will regulate. She'll usually sleep for four to six hours at a time, going to bed fairly late and waking early. If you feed her just prior to bedtime, night-feedings will decrease.

At three to four months, her daytime sleep habits will also become more consistent. This is when most children start adopting a regular sleep pattern, and parents can begin enjoying some uninterrupted rest. They also generally take two or three naps per day—a good time for you to nap, too. If your child wakes during the night outside of regular feeding times, check on her *silently*, with the lights off, and don't pick her up. Sometimes, all she needs is to see you're there, especially when separation anxiety peaks between five and ten months.

At nine months, night feedings usually cease (say "Hallelujah!" sister) as does the third nap. The morning nap will eventually disappear between twelve and twenty-one months, at which time an earlier bedtime may help to ensure your child is getting enough sleep. Hopefully an earlier bedtime for her means an earlier bedtime for you, so the whole family can be happy and well rested.

Should I let my child sleep in my bed?

This is a family decision. In about two-thirds of countries, children sleep with their parents until age three or four. In the US and other industrialized nations, about one-third of urban white families and two-thirds of African-American families sleep together for all or part of the night.

If you decide to co-sleep, keep in mind cultural and social norms; after your child is about three to four years old, it may be best for him to sleep independently in order to avoid teasing and develop his own sleep skills. Transitioning your child to his own bed is usually not difficult if the whole family is well rested. And if after that age your child continues to have bad dreams every once in a while and wants to crawl into bed with you, go ahead and let him on some occasions. Just don't let it become a habit. If you need help getting him to sleep in his own bed, refer to the approaches at the end of this chapter for calming child fears.

How much reading and TV should I allow prior to bed?

Sharing a story with your child at night or, if he's old enough, allowing him to read by himself is important to educational development and a great part of any bedtime routine. If, however, the little guy starts staying up late reading Harry Potter, then some rules are in order. Set a time or chapter limit, or else allow him to go to bed earlier for more reading time.

Television is different, though. Don't let your child watch TV within an hour of bedtime. Children with TVs in their room go to sleep later and get significantly less rest than other kids. Problems that arise include fears/nightmares, trouble sleeping caused by over-stimulation from lights/colors on the screen (even if it's a relatively calm show), "needing" TV to fall asleep, viewing inappropriate shows due to less parental supervision, childhood obesity, and less family time. Set a good example by taking the TV out of your own room. If there are complaints of "I'll miss my favorite show!" invest in a DVR. The same rules go for all electronics—keep the computer, Nintendo DS, Xbox, GameCube, Wii, iPod, iPad, and (heaven forbid) the cell phone out of your child's room. As a general rule of thumb, if it was invented after the eighties take it out!

How can I protect my child from SIDS and other nighttime risks?

Knowing your child is safe at night will help you and her sleep peacefully. Sudden Infant Death Syndrome (SIDS) is a major concern of new parents. But its risk has been cut in half since the American Academy of Pediatrics began recommending that babies be laid on their backs rather than on their stomachs. Contrary to popular belief, this will not cause permanent deformities such as a flat head. Note that when your baby is old enough to roll over by herself (generally between four and seven months), she is past the highest-risk stage for SIDS.

Safe Slumber Tips

- Put baby to sleep on his back
- Avoid soft bedding, bulky comforters, pillows, and large stuffed toys
- Dress him in a warm, one-piece sleeper
- Use just one thin blanket, tucked into the crib sides
- Set the room temperature at 65–70°F
- Keep the crib away from windows and radiators
- Use a firm mattress that fits snugly against the crib walls
- Lock the crib rails and keep their tops at least 26 inches above the mattress (higher as baby learns to stand)
- Make sure the crib bars are no more than 2 3/8 inches apart
- Make the baby's room a no-pet zone
- For head-bangers/thrashers, swaddle or use crib bumpers until baby can safely pull himself up
- Never leave your child alone with a bottle at night (it causes tooth decay)

Should I get up when he starts crying or let him "cry it out"?

If something is causing your child genuine pain or distress, don't ignore it. But if his sobs are "protest crying," then most experts recommend not soothing him.

Protest crying includes refusing to go to bed or not wanting to be left alone. Between five and ten months of age, it often stems from normal separation anxiety, but after that it's usually just the child trying to assert himself. For younger kids, use the Check/Reassure

> ### *Coping with a Crybaby*
>
> If you attend to every whimper, you'll encourage sleep-fragmentation (lack of continuous sleep), insomnia, and the belief that crying is a good way to get Mom's attention. This is why baby monitors are not always a good idea. They can encourage parents to attend to every cry rather than the few that mean hunger or strong separation anxiety. Trust us: you'll hear those!

Approach. Quietly check on him every five minutes or so until he falls asleep. These visits will reassure him that you're there and that he's safe. Keep the visits brief, don't turn on the lights, be quiet, and avoid picking him up so as not to encourage more of it. Even if he cries for hours on end, stick with this strategy. Otherwise, if you give in and pick him up, he'll learn that he can "win." If the crying is driving you crazy now, imagine how you'll feel when it becomes habitual.

Naps are different, though. Don't let your child cry for a long time after putting him in for a nap. Because naps are only one to two hours long, extended intervals of crying will take up almost half or all of the nap. So, if your child cries at naptime, start out by using the same Check/Reassure Approach detailed earlier, but if an hour passes with no success, it's okay to take him out of bed and enjoy quiet time instead.

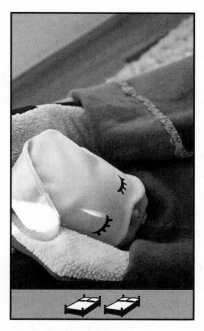

Downtime Organic Sleepytime Mask helps children learn that closing their eyes is one step in falling asleep. The closed eyelashes that detail the flip-down mask let others know not to disturb baby's sleep.

Some parents struggle with this whole "cry-it-out" concept because they can't stand doing nothing. The truth is you're not doing "nothing"; you're helping your child develop independent sleep skills that will ensure healthful rest habits later in life. You can also take comfort in the fact that emotional problems do not develop from parents ignoring protest crying.

Calm Your Early Bird

If your child consistently wakes up too early, investigate what's causing it. Is his room too cold? Turn up the heat. Is there a loud garbage truck? Put a fan or radio tuned to white noise in his room. Does a stream of light wake him up? Close or darken the shades. If the early waking is natural, encourage your child to play quietly in his room until a specified time ("When the clock says 7-0-0, you can come wake up Mommy"), or try an *earlier* bedtime (which surprisingly leads to sleeping *later*).

Every night it's a struggle to put my child to bed. Any tips for making it easier?

Fifty-two percent of preschoolers and 42 percent of school-age children stall at bedtime. Why do they do it? The list is long: child temperament, sleep environment, poor sleep schedule/ habits, sleep deprivation, fears, or conflicting parenting styles ("But Daddy lets me stay up and watch *Monday Night Football!*").

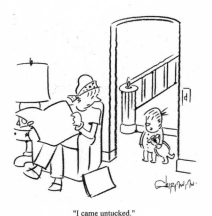

"I came untucked."

Here are some things you can try to discourage curtain calls and other bedtime stall tactics:

- *Be consistent.* Keep to a regular, age-appropriate sleep schedule and a consistent bedtime routine.

- *Establish clear rules.* Bath at 7, quiet reading time at 7:30, then lights out by 8. It may even be helpful to write these rules out and post them in the child's room.

> **No Toys-R-Us or Time-Out Town**
>
> To help your child stay in bed at night, try changing the way he thinks about his bedroom. Don't make it a playland of toys and games, and don't use it as his designated time-out spot. This could lead him to associate his bedroom with playtime or being in trouble.

- *Fade the bedtime.* If your child is particularly difficult, start with a later bedtime (when she's *really* tired), then move it up a bit each night until you reach the desired time.

- *Leave her alone.* Falling asleep independently (and going back to sleep after waking up at night) is a *learned* process. You can begin to teach your child this at a very young age by placing her in the crib when she's drowsy and leaving the room while she's still awake. Don't let it get to the point where she *needs* you there to fall asleep.

- *Use transitional objects.* If your child is older, encourage her to sleep with something that brings her comfort such as a blanket, stuffed animal, or even a piece of clothing that smells like Mom or Dad (well, maybe not Dad).

- *Provide positive reinforcement.* Reward your child for following bedtime rules and staying tucked-in at night. Give her a sticker for every successful night and, when she earns ten, award her a small prize or privilege. And praise her for her cooperation.

- *Respond when necessary.* Don't ignore reasonable nighttime requests for drinks of water or bathroom visits, but fulfill them in a brief and matter-of-fact way. If your child gets out of bed, let her see that there's nothing exciting going on before silently and unemotionally returning her to bed.

- *Fade the door.* If your child's getting out of bed too often and she normally sleeps with the door open, try "fading the door." Put tape marks on the floor, and each time she gets out of bed, move the door to the next mark (closer to being shut). Chances are she will choose staying in bed over letting her door shut all the way.

Help! He says there's a monster in his closet!

Preschoolers have incredible imaginations. Their creativity can lead to nighttime fears, nightmares, and reluctance to stay in bed. Some things that encourage these fears are sleep-deprivation, exposure to scary things on the Internet or TV, and stress from life events such as potty training or a new sibling. Fortunately, there are several approaches that can be used individually or in combination that will help your child sleep more pleasantly:

1. *Discuss* her fear with her during the day and reassure her of being safe at night.
2. *Explain* that monsters are not real, but at the same time admit that you get scared sometimes too, and explain how you deal with a fear. Reward and praise her for her braveness.
3. *Change* the way she thinks about nighttime by playing an in-the-dark game (during the day), such as hide-and-seek or flashlight tag (in a darkened room). You can also try to teach her some very basic relaxation techniques, such as deep breathing, which will help calm her if the fear returns.

In all cases, it may be helpful to keep your child's bedroom door slightly open or use a nightlight.

Developing good sleep habits in youngsters is absolutely critical.

A study at Johns Hopkins Bloomberg School of Public Health concluded that less sleep can increase a child's risk of being overweight or obese by as much as 92 percent, compared to kids getting adequate sleep. If your children aren't meeting recommendations (see chart), set some rules. Every additional hour of sleep will reduce their risk of becoming obese by 9 percent.

Age	Recommended Hours
10 years	At least 9 hours
5-10 years	At least 10 hours
Under 5 years	At least 11 hours

Perhaps the best thing you can do for your youngsters is to become a good role model as far as sleep. If you value sleep, your child will pick up on that too.

10 Teenage Walking Zombies

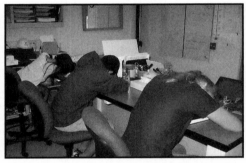

80 percent of teens are sleep-deprived, and 43 percent feel sleepy all day.

Parents, this chapter is specifically designed for your teenagers and their unique sleep needs. It is particularly challenging for adolescents to stay well rested, but it's absolutely vital that they do so in order to grow up healthy, stay out of trouble, and excel. Read this chapter first for some valuable insight, and then suggest they read it too.

Attention teenagers!

Do you often feel sleepy during class? Do you go to the library or computer lab and instantly fall asleep? Do you stress about good grades, getting into college, landing a good job, or that ever-present, vague, and anxiety-ridden notion adults call "your future"? Do you experiment with drugs, tobacco, and alcohol or feel peer pressure to do so? Do you ever feel like the hours you invest in academics and sports don't pay off with better performance? Are your eye-lids drooping right now?

If so, and if you feel you may not be living up to your potential, the reason could be the quantity

> "What we consider the negative aspects of adolescence—rebellion, violence, drug abuse, dropping out—are caused by or exaggerated by sleep deprivation."
> —*William Dement, MD*

and quality of your sleep. Get comfortable and continue reading because we're about to not only answer all your questions about sleep during this unique stage of your life, but we're also going to show you how to have more energy, get better grades, be a more successful athlete, and even have a more rewarding social life. You have no idea the sparkling person you can be.

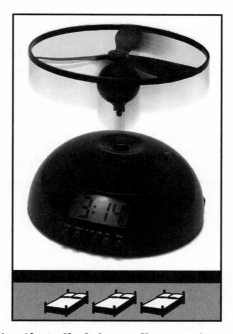

This ***Flying Alarm Clock*** shoots off a rotor when it goes off. The alarm will not shut off until you get out of bed, find the rotor, and replace it!

Wonder why you're always so tired?

There's a battle raging inside your body. On one side, your need for sleep increases at puberty. At the same time, you experience a growth hormone spurt from puberty until age twenty-five that not only determines your physical development but also, unfortunately, extends your natural period of wakefulness.

According to Dr. Charles Czeisler at Harvard University, the teenage brain is biologically set to fall asleep at 3:00 AM and begin to awaken sometime after 11:00 AM. As a result, 80 percent of teens do not get enough sleep, and 43 percent say they feel sleepy all day. One test: if you need an alarm clock to wake up, you're not getting adequate sleep.

What difference does it make if I'm sleep-deprived?

You've probably been tired for so long, you don't remember what it's like to be wide awake. You may be unaware of how diminished alertness compromises all aspects of life. Think of it this way: sleep is food for your brain. If your brain doesn't have enough nourishment, it's not going to be able to perform at a high level. During sleep, essential body functions take place that are critical for your growth, performance, and general well-being. Here's a rundown:

> **More z's = less lbs.**
>
> Increasing your sleep by one hour is the best diet. You can lose as much as a pound a week just by sleeping a little longer.

Emotional: Without sleep, you get moody. You snip at your friends and parents. You're more vulnerable to irritability, anxiety, and depression.

Physical: Sleep six hours or less each night, and you've raised your susceptibility to viral infection by 50 percent compared to those getting adequate rest. In one experiment, when cold germs were sprayed into the nasal passage of six-hour sleepers, they caught colds. But when eight-hour sleepers were exposed to the same germs, they stayed healthy. You're likely to gain weight, too. A six-hour sleeper is 23 percent more likely to be obese than an eight or nine-hour sleeper.

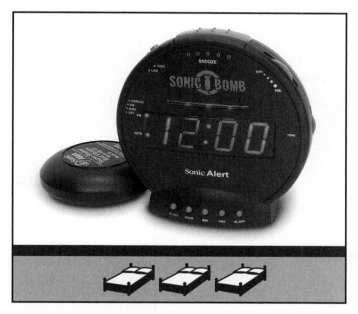

Teenagers are notoriously difficult to wake up. **Sonic Bomb Clock** has an adjustable volume alarm with a maximum loudness of 113 decibels (a jackhammer is 100 decibels!) It also vibrates. Slip it under your mattress and you'll be shaken up.

Athletic: Sleepiness impairs reaction time, awareness, and motor skills. Athletes who forego early-morning workouts and practice only in the afternoon perform better due to the extra sleep.

Mental: According to Jennifer C. Cousins, a postdoctoral fellow at the University of Pittsburgh Medical Center, better quality sleep and more efficient sleep may lead to higher grades, especially in math.

The sleep-deprived are more prone to drowsiness, nodding off at inappropriate times, and microsleeps. These are short bouts of subconscious sleep lasting up to ninety seconds of which you are unaware. Remember that the next time you're driving home late at night. Teenagers cause 50 percent of all driving accidents although they represent far less than half of the driving population.

Without adequate sleep, your alertness, concentration, memory, productivity, perception, senses, and ability to think critically and creatively and to multitask are all significantly impaired. It's also difficult to assimilate and analyze new information and communicate effectively. Ironically, these are the skills you need in order to manage and balance an increase in homework, social activities, and everyday stressors.

Mary Carskadon at Brown University found that students who slept 17-33 minutes more than their peers each night increased their performance by an entire letter grade. Adolescents who sleep 9 hours have significantly better grades than those who sleep 6, have fewer learning difficulties and are tardy less often. A sleep study of 450 students at Cornell by Maas, Fortgang, Driscoll and Robbins, using the Zeo instrument as an objective measurement of sleep

> **New finding: From zzz's to A's!**
>
> Students who receive A's and B's in school report going to bed earlier and getting more sleep than students with lower grades. A recent study at Cornell University found students who sleep 9 hours have significantly better grades than those who sleep 6.

length and quality, found a significant correlation between total amount of sleep and academic performance, and an even more significant correlation between grades and amount of deep sleep. The worst sleepers (in the lowest quartile of the study) after being taught the rules of good sleep hygiene, increased their sleep length by 90 minutes and their sleep efficiency by 30 percent. Students struggling or failing in school (getting grades ranging from C to F) obtain about 25 minutes less sleep and go to bed an average of 40 minutes later on school nights than students getting A and B marks. They also report more variation in weeknight versus weekend sleep schedules. Although it is difficult to isolate causation in these assessments, the evidence does suggest that sleep deprivation is strongly associated with lower academic performance.

Can't I just make up for lost sleep on the weekends?

Any additional sleep is helpful, but sleeping until noon on Saturday and Sunday is not the best way to recover what was lost during the week. In fact, such a yo-yo sleep schedule will throw your internal clock even more out of whack. Sure, you stay up late on Fridays and Saturdays to hang with friends and then sleep it off for half the next day, but when Sunday night rolls around (and it always does), if you try to force yourself to sleep at 10:00 or 11:00 PM, you just won't be tired enough. So you toss and turn and fall asleep at 2:00 AM, making it an ugly battle to get out of bed the next morning. You go to school with the Monday-morning blahs, having given yourself eastbound jetlag without ever leaving your hometown.

How important is it to maintain a regular sleep-wake schedule?

Regularity of sleep is almost as important as quantity of sleep. If you stay up late on Friday and Saturday nights and sleep in the next morning, you'll be far more tired during the week, even if you go to bed at a reasonable hour. We're not recommending skipping special events in order to get your nine hours, but do try your best to maintain a regular sleep-wake schedule. You have one biological clock; not one for the school week and one for the weekend. You must synchronize the hours you spend in bed with the sleepy phase on that clock.

The best thing you can do right now is to avoid losing sleep in the future. Count back 9.25 hours from the time you must get up and use that as your regular bedtime. It will take a few weeks to get synchronized, so be patient. Making this permanent change to your sleep-wake schedule and sticking to it Monday through Monday, will actually *change* your life!

Do drugs and alcohol compound the effects of sleep deprivation?

As mentioned previously, in terms of your ability to drive a car, one drink on six hours of sleep (what you're likely getting) is the equivalent of having six drinks on eight hours of sleep. Never get into a car if the driver is even the least bit sleep-deprived and has been drinking. It's an accident waiting to happen. Sleep deprivation has a similar interaction with drugs such as marijuana.

How many hours of sleep do I need?

For full alertness, you need 9.25 hours of sleep every night. You can do it! Make sleep a priority, and you'll start seeing the benefits within two or three days. You might think there's not enough time in the day to get everything done, let alone get nine hours of sack time, but you'll quickly notice that being in a better mood and being more aware makes you more efficient and effective during the day. Believe it or not, you'll be able to wake up without an alarm clock. You'll get more done and still have time left over.

When should I go to bed?

Melatonin, the body's natural sleep-enhancing hormone, is secreted later in the evening among teens, so it may be difficult for you to nod off before 11:00 PM. Nonetheless, try to go to bed as early as naturally possible. Establishing a pre-bed ritual and sticking to that routine can trick your body into feeling sleepier. For instance, take a warm shower, keep the lights low, do some easy stretching or listen to soft, classical music. No heavy metal, head-banger ballads within an hour of bedtime.

(For tips on pre-bed rituals, see Chapter 6 on successful strategies so you can *Sleep for Success!*).

What about napping?

If you're starved for sleep, take a twenty-minute restorative nap after school. If you nap any longer than this, you will wake up groggy and might not be able to get to sleep on time that night. Napping will help make up for lost sleep, and it'll generally enable you to get through the rest of the day and evening without additional drowsiness or nocturnal insomnia.

> "For time-strapped teens, something has got to go. I feel very strongly that the first thing to go should be an after-school job. Allowing or encouraging after-school jobs is actually an irresponsible attitude toward school and health habits on the part of parents."
> —William C. Dement, MD

What role does caffeine play in all of this?

We all respond to caffeine differently since body weight plays a factor. However, too much caffeine will affect your ability to fall asleep and get quality rest. The general rule is to limit caffeine consumption to 150mg per day and to avoid all caffeinated beverages and chocolate after 2:00 PM. Many teens try to "power study" by drinking a Red Bull or other highly caffeinated beverage in the evening and then cramming into the wee hours of the morning. You won't retain the studied material for long, though, and might very well sleep through an alarm before your exam. Several of our students have

> *Know Your Limits:* Recommended maximum daily consumption of caffeine for teens is 150 mg
>
> 8oz cup of coffee = 100 mg
> 8oz cup of tea = 50 mg
> 1oz dark chocolate = 20 mg
> Red Bull = 80 mg

experienced this—even in a class that focuses on sleep research. How embarrassing.☹

Do you see the light?

Sunlight regulates your internal clock. Expose yourself to bright daylight-spectrum lighting, either sunlight or artificial lamps, as soon as you wake up. Doing so, for even as little as fifteen minutes, will tell your brain that it should be up and at 'em. Conversely, keep the lights low before bedtime. Especially avoid having high-intensity halogen lamps in your bedroom.

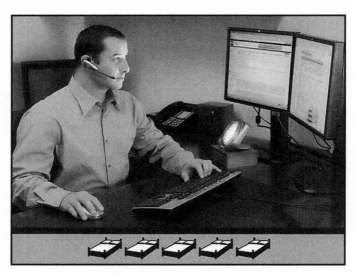

Wake up to *LiteBook!* With fifty LED daylight spectrum lights, a fifteen-minute exposure to this gadget has a similar effect as one to two shots of caffeine—without the side effects.

Is it true that after-school jobs are associated with poor sleep?

Yes. Although 55 percent of American teens work after school, these part-time jobs have been linked with less sleep time, more falling asleep in class, and more oversleeping. It's interesting to note that after-school jobs typically aren't providing funds for college but rather for entertainment and luxury items. Don't squander your chance for getting into a great college. The extra time spent on academics just might be your edge in getting a college scholarship.

How can I convince my school that early classes are unreasonable?

Time and again, objective studies show that later school-start times actually improve students' well-being and performance as well as reduce illness, accidents, and the use of stimulants and drugs. It is a common misperception that later school-start times entice teens to stay up later at night. This is not the case.

Case in point: The administration at Deerfield Academy, a preparatory school in Massachusetts, established earlier check-in times at night and later class-start times in the morning. This pilot program gave students an extra hour of rest. The results have been overwhelmingly positive:

> "The effects have been immediate and dramatic. We will continue to address the importance of sleep on a day-to-day basis. We are never going back to our former schedule."
> —*Margarita Curtis, head of school, Deerfield Academy*

- Grades rose to a record winter-term high

- Athletic records improved

- Seventeen percent more hot breakfasts were consumed.

- Teachers reported students showed increased alertness, readiness to engage, and better mood in morning classes.

- Visits to the health center were also down 20 percent in a year when other schools reported substantial increases in the flu and colds.

I'm never going to be able to follow your advice. I'm just too busy.

It may seem difficult to turn off the lights, especially at 11:00 PM when you still have a ton of homework and all your friends are texting you, but trust us and try it. After sixteen hours, the quality of your work is essentially worthless anyway. You'll be in a better mood while being more efficient, effective, and productive. You'll eventually find it easier to get everything accomplished *and* get adequate sleep.

If good intentions aren't enough, consider cutting back on the activities you're involved in. According to a study released by the Kaiser Family Foundation, eight to eighteen-year-olds devote an average of seven hours and thirty-eight minutes (7:38) to using entertainment media across a typical day. This amounts to more than fifty-three hours a week, a tremendous sleep thief.

Dear Dr. Maas,

Thank you for your powerful presentation at Deerfield Academy. From that day on, I have generally succeeded in securing nine hours (or at least eight and a half) of sleep for myself every night. Before, I was sleeping around seven hours a night.

My life has changed dramatically. I wake up cheerful and looking forward to the day. I am far less anxious and cranky with my friends and parents. In school, I have managed to accomplish more than ever even with fewer waking hours. My grades are the highest I've ever had, even though I'm taking all honors/AP courses this year. I can practically recite my history textbook when, before, I wasn't able to retain most of what I read. In general, I can focus better and read more quickly and efficiently. [And I have] more time to spend with my friends and family than I did in the past.

I don't intend to brag, but only to explain the transformation I have experienced and express my deepest gratitude for your work. This simple adjustment has changed my life: it has made me happier and uncovered a range of opportunities I had never imagined.

Thank you!

A.C.D.

Sleep should be a priority at your age, because it sets the tone for the rest of your life. Besides, not getting enough rest is probably affecting your ability to excel at the extracurriculars that are affecting your sleep schedule. It's a vicious cycle that is up to you to break.

If you follow all the guidelines for getting better sleep, you are likely to see a significant change in your grades, your athletic ability, your health, and your happiness. Be patient. It takes teens two to three weeks of good sleep to reach maximum potential. What are you waiting for? Start today!

11

Challenges for the Elderly

"Retiring" in Style

No, this chapter isn't about how to rebuild a 401K or find a bargain condo in Boca. It's about ensuring a far more important part of the twilight years—your health and happiness. Sleep woes plague the elderly. In the next few pages, we'll discuss how to overcome the most common problems and retire in style (if only for the night). But first, are you or a loved one:

- Over age 65?

- Having more difficulty falling asleep than in middle age?

- Waking up several times during the night?

- Waking up too early in the morning?

- Needing a long nap in the afternoon?

Good sleep helps us stay younger longer. With age comes change, however, and so it is with certain elements of sleep. Although there's no evidence that the need for sleep is any different in seniors than in middle-age adults, the ability to sleep does diminish. It becomes more difficult to sleep for long periods due to changes in the brain (hardening of the arteries), health woes, and common medications (particularly those taken for hypertension, Type II diabetes, and rheumatoid arthritis). Additionally, there's often anxiety over losing loved ones, living on a fixed income, or just getting old. The sad truth is that seniors report more sleep problems than any other segment of the population. But, like deteriorating eyesight and hearing, poor sleep doesn't have to be an unavoidable part of aging. Knowing what causes the problems and how to address them can enable anyone of any age to sleep like a baby.

> **Why Grandma is Always Knitting**—
> Ever wonder why elderly people keep their homes so warm or wear sweaters in July? Adults who suffer from insomnia don't detect temperature change very well. What's more, a bedroom that's too hot or too cool (but unnoticed) could be causing (or perpetuating) the insomnia. Experts suggest a hot bath before bed to raise skin temperature, lower core body temperature, and encourage drowsiness. (But check with your doctor to be sure that's safe for you—and Grandma.)

How does the ability to sleep change with age?

Seniors often shake their heads and say, "What I wouldn't give to sleep as soundly as I did when I was young." Unfortunately, once we get into our thirties we tend to lose some function in the cerebral cortex. This area of the brain plays a key role in initiating sleep.

Aside from this change, the amount of deep, slow-wave sleep we typically experience decreases with age. As this important sleep stage dwindles, so do levels of human growth hormone (HGH). Women, however, secrete more of their HGH during the day so they're not as negatively affected by the loss of deep, slow-wave sleep, which often accompanies the onset of menopause.

Dr. Eve Van Cauter of the University of Chicago reports a decrease in REM sleep, particularly in men over age fifty. REM sleep is the stage that regulates production of the stress hormone cortisol. During the evening, when cortisol levels should bottom out, this hormone is instead elevated, causing a state of heightened awareness that makes it harder to fall asleep.

It's important to note that healthy seniors with good bedtime habits report little to no sleep problems, even though their rest is generally lighter and more fragmented than younger individuals. In fact, older Americans who sleep well may actually sleep better than eighteen to fifty-four-year-olds. It's proof that sleeping worse doesn't have to be a natural consequence of getting old.

What are the most common sleep problems among the elderly?

Sixty-seven percent of older adults report having one or more of the following problems at least a few times per week:

- *Difficulty falling asleep.* Thirteen percent of men and 36 percent of women over age sixty-five report taking longer than thirty minutes to fall asleep. This is probably due to a decrease in the amount of melatonin the brain secretes with age. (Melatonin is the calming hormone that essentially tucks us in each night.)

- *Waking repeatedly, or waking up early and not being able to fall back to sleep.* Also known as "sleep maintenance insomnia," this is common in the elderly. It can have many causes, including breathing disorders and leg jerks during sleep, depression, chronic pain, heartburn, side effects from medications, circadian rhythm disturbances, or just a poor sleep environment.

- *Snoring or repetitive pauses in breathing.* Undiagnosed sleep apnea occurs in 4 percent of males and 2 percent of females under age sixty-five. But once over that age, the percentages rise to 26 percent and 24 percent, respectively. Sleep apnea is a huge contributor to daytime drowsiness among the elderly. (See Chapter 17 for a more detailed discussion of sleep disorders.)

- *Periodic limb movements.* The National Sleep Foundation reports that about 35 percent of people age sixty-five and older experience periodic limb movements during sleep— repetitive motions that usually affect the legs and happen every twenty to forty seconds. Sometimes they're muscle twitches, jerking movements, or an upward flexing of the foot. Although not considered medically severe, they can be a primary factor in chronic insomnia and daytime fatigue because they prevent sound sleep.

- *Restless legs syndrome (RLS).* The National Institute of Neurological Disorders and Strokes describes RLS as unpleasant sensations in the legs and an uncontrollable urge to move when at rest in order to relieve them. These sensations are described as burning, creeping, tugging, or like insects crawling inside the legs. Often called paresthesias (abnormal sensations) or dysesthesias (unpleasant abnormal sensations), these symptoms can range from uncomfortable to irritating to painful. The most distinctive or unusual aspect of the condition is that lying down and trying to relax activates the symptoms. As a result, most people with RLS have difficulty falling asleep and staying asleep. Left untreated, the condition causes exhaustion. Many people with RLS report that their jobs, personal relationships, and routine daily activities are strongly affected. They're often unable to concentrate, remember things, or accomplish daily tasks.

How do other age-related conditions affect sleep quality?

The healthier you are, the better you'll sleep, regardless of age. Conversely, the more medical concerns you have, the more likely you'll have problems sleeping. Seniors who report four or more medical conditions (i.e., high blood pressure, arthritis, memory problems, heart disease, diabetes, cancer, depression) are more likely to sleep less than six hours per night, experience daytime drowsiness, and suffer from sleep disorders than those with fewer or no medical conditions. Plus, older adults with positive moods and outlooks, as well as more active and engaged lifestyles (i.e., exercising, volunteering, and having someone to speak with about problems) are more likely to sleep seven to nine hours and have fewer nighttime complaints.

> According to Michael Irwin, MD, UCLA, sleep disturbance is associated with declines in health and with increases in depression and all causes of mortality in older adults.

- *Alzheimer's* and other forms of dementia often disrupt and fragment sleep. As a result, sufferers can be so tired during the day that they drift in and out of consciousness, often for an hour at a time. Not being able to stay asleep at night also literally opens the door for late-night wandering—something that's disruptive to everyone involved and potentially life-threatening.

- *Arthritis, back trouble, and other pain-related conditions* can affect sleep by making it uncomfortable to lie down or be immobile for any length of time. Make sure your mattress is right for you—be it foam, waterbed, air or traditional inner spring. For many people living with arthritis and chronic back pain, a good mattress is the difference between frustrating, fragmented sleep and restorative, healing rest.

- *Heart trouble* often causes shortness of breath, especially when the person is prone. This disturbs sleep, promotes daytime drowsiness and pushes up blood pressure, all of which compound the condition.

- *Depression* can make falling asleep a challenge because the body is under emotional stress. What's more, adults over age sixty with a history of depression and who are suffering from disturbed sleep are at greater risk for a relapse. Not only can depression affect our sleep for the worse, our sleep (if we don't make a conscious effort to regulate it) can worsen our depression.

Is it smart for seniors to nap?

Healthy, active seniors with good bedtime habits, who have no trouble sleeping at night, can nap whenever they feel the need. But not surprisingly, such individuals are the least likely to doze during the day because they're well rested in the first place.

There's some interesting research, though, showing that older women who nap daily are 44 percent more likely to die earlier than those who don't nap. Even older women who reported napping just three or more hours per week had a significantly greater risk of death. Now, before you call to check on Grandma, understand that it's unlikely napping itself is to blame. Rather, the drowsiness attributed to daily and extended napping in seniors is usually an indication of a serious underlying sleep or medical problem, and addressing it usually reduces mortality risk. So if you or an older member of your family is feeling sleepy all day, consult a doctor immediately to find out if something else might be to blame.

So what's the best advice for seniors who want to sleep through the night?

Being older does not exempt you from needing to set the stage for sleep.

Follow all the strategies for better sleep habits outlined in Chapter 6. But if that still doesn't work, here are some additional alternatives:

> **New finding:** Practicing tai chi, a 2,000–year-old martial art known for its gentle, flowing movements, can facilitate sleep in older adults. Researchers at UCLA found that over a twenty-five-week period, adults who practiced twenty simple tai chi moves showed improved sleep quality and less daytime drowsiness (compared to a control group). Those who practiced tai chi also rated their own sleep quality better.

- *Listen to light classical music on low volume at bedtime.* This can increase the length and depth of sleep in the elderly by as much as 35 percent. Make sure the music turns off automatically so it won't awaken you when you reach lighter stages of sleep later.

- *Limit your time in bed.* Some seniors are so worried about getting eight hours of sleep that they go to bed too early and stay there for ten to twelve hours, hoping that somehow they'll manage to get at least eight. Bad idea. It sounds paradoxical for an insomniac, but if you're struggling to get to sleep, try going to bed much later than usual one night. In fact, force yourself to stay awake as long as possible but keep your waking time constant. This method of "sleep restriction" ensures that when you finally let yourself go to bed, you'll be so tired that you'll fall right into a deep, efficient slumber. After you've seen some success with this approach, move up your bedtime by twenty to thirty minutes each night until you're sleeping pretty much through the night. Be patient, though—it can take several weeks to establish a regular and adequate sleep schedule.

- *Don't count sheep.* If you can't stay asleep, get out of bed, keep the lights low, and go into another room to read or listen to music. Do anything that puts your mind at ease. Only go back to bed when you start feeling drowsy again.

- *Don't obsess about getting up repeatedly to pee.* Of course, talk to your doctor if the problem is severe, but keep in mind that the body's ability to "hold it" diminishes naturally with age. What's not normal is being unable to fall back to sleep within ten minutes. To minimize disturbances, drink less water and alcohol in the three hours before bed, and when you do get up keep the lights low. (And remember to put down the seat, will you?)

Should seniors take sleeping pills?

Prescription sleeping pills work, no doubt about it. But for the elderly, the risks associated with such medication significantly outweigh the benefits. These pills don't let you experience the normal ins, outs, ups, and downs of natural, restorative sleep, so you derive very few advantages. Plus, they increase the risk of accidents such as falls and car crashes as much as twofold. Even milder, over-the-counter (OTC) sleeping pills can cause complications for senior citizens, depending on what other medications they're taking and what specific medical conditions they have. If you're considering using *any* sleep aid, no matter how "mild," it's best to thoroughly discuss it with a doctor beforehand. Sometimes OTC sleep-inducing medications can alleviate symptoms that make it difficult to get comfortable in bed,

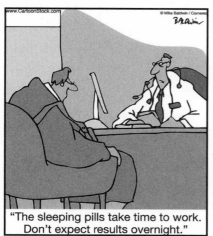

"The sleeping pills take time to work. Don't expect results overnight."

but a good rule of thumb is to not add any pills to your daily regimen until you've discussed it thoroughly with your physician.

No matter what, realize that simply because you aren't as young as you used to be doesn't mean you can't *Sleep for Success!*

12

Women & Sleep

Hostage to Hormones

For women, sleep is routinely interrupted by fluctuating hormones, unique life challenges, night-time child care, anxiety, and sometimes even depression (especially after giving birth or just before menopause). In fact, 56 percent of women can't seem to get a good night's sleep. Is it an inevitable part of the feminine mystique? Or is there something women are doing wrong?

Are men and women really that different when it comes to sleep?

Yes, men are from Mars and women are from Venus when it comes to how much sleep they get and the resulting consequences. Maybe that's no surprise given the huge percentage of women who hold two jobs: one outside the home and one inside.

Some facts:

- Women generally need more sleep than men to be fully alert during the day.

- Twenty-four percent more women than men report having insomnia at least a few nights per week.

- Women complain more often about getting poor or less-restorative sleep than men.

- Fifty percent more women than men say drowsiness negatively affects their daily tasks.

- Thirty-two percent of women use sleeping pills (versus 21 percent of men).

- Women complain more about being awakened during the night by others, like children and snoring partners.

- Eighty-six percent of women say their husbands snore, and more than half claim it disrupts their sleep. (Comparatively, 57 percent of men report that their wives snore and only 15 percent are bothered by it.)

What affects a woman's sleep most?

Over half of the sleep problems women deal with stem from hormonal changes. Natural fluctuations in testosterone, cortisol, and melatonin levels can all disrupt sleep, especially during menstruation, pregnancy, and at the start of menopause.

How does the menstrual cycle impact sleep?

In women of childbearing age, 70 percent experience disrupted sleep for two and a half days during the premenstrual period. During menstruation, most hormone levels drop, as does metabolic rate, which causes poor sleep and excessive daytime drowsiness. Specifically, during the early luteal phase of the menstrual cycle (days fifteen to seventeen, assuming a twenty-eight-day cycle) body temperature increases, thus lengthening the time it takes to fall asleep and also decreasing the depth of sleep. In the late luteal phase (days twenty-four to twenty-eight), estrogen and progesterone levels fall, causing frequent night-time awakenings.

How does pregnancy affect sleep?

During pregnancy, 80 percent of women report having more disrupted sleep than usual. And 60 percent say the sleep they get is not refreshing (probably due again to shifting hormone levels). The frequent need to urinate, plus backaches, heartburn, nausea, vomiting, nightmares, leg cramps, baby movements, and, of course, those irresistible cravings for chocolate-cake donuts, certainly don't help the situation.

In the first trimester, expectant mothers often experience excessive daytime sleepiness because increased progesterone secretion disrupts nocturnal rest. Sleep often improves during the second trimester, even though women at this stage have less deep sleep, more awakenings, and may begin to suffer from restless legs syndrome. The third trimester tends to affect sleep the most because of the dramatic change in hormones, the girth of the body, the inability to get comfortable, and, in some cases, sleep apnea. Some women hardly sleep at all very close to giving birth.

How can I sleep better during my pregnancy?

Because sleep is so crucial to your developing baby, talk with your doctor if you're having difficulty getting adequate rest. Taking naps, especially in the early afternoon, is a good way to ensure that over a twenty-four-hour period you come close to getting the amount of sleep you

Women, more so than men, use cigarettes to relieve stress and relax. But, nicotine actually stimulates the brain and other bodily functions, making sleep more difficult. It's one more reason to quit.

need. Remember, sleep is cumulative. To get more comfortable, try putting a pillow between your knees while lying in bed (to take the strain off your back and reduce pain); eat your main meal at midday in order to avoid night-time indigestion and eat small-but-frequent meals the rest of the time; and avoid spicy foods, acidic fruit juices, and alcohol.

Some women find they sleep better if they elevate their head, or even if they sleep in a recliner. Experiment with positions until you find the one that's most comfortable for you. When lying down, try resting on your left side to increase blood flow. Learning a few relaxation techniques, such as meditation, can also be helpful in preparing the body and mind for sleep.

What about after the baby's born: how much sleep can a new mom expect to lose?

If there are no complications for mother and baby, it's possible that sleep can return to normal fairly quickly after childbirth. But, as any parent knows, this is more theory than fact. Primary caregivers can expect to lose up to seven hundred hours of sleep in their baby's first year of life. That's nearly two hours per night. This can be exacerbated if a new mother suffers from major postpartum depression, as 10 percent to 15 percent of moms do.

What happens to a woman's sleep pattern when she reaches middle age?

Twenty percent of middle-aged women sleep less than six hours per night, compared to 12 percent of younger women. This is likely due to a combination of things, such as stress, depressed mood, or physiological symptoms like chronic pain. At this life stage, women often find themselves not only worrying about their children, their relationship, and their career, but also their aging parents. They are consumed by the commonly shared feeling that "there aren't enough hours in the day." Women can also become depressed about their fading youth and the onset of age-related health problems. Not surprisingly, all of this can keep one up at night.

In what way does menopause affect sleep?

At the onset of menopause, 66 percent of women complain of difficulty falling asleep and staying asleep. Menopausal women are also more likely to keep getting up to go to the bathroom. Forty-four percent experience hot flashes at night so severe that their sleep is disrupted.

When you were younger, the bedtime "hots" was something quite different (and a lot more enjoyable) than what you're experiencing now. (And if you're overweight and/or smoke, you're making them even worse.) Unfortunately, there aren't many long-term studies on the use of natural remedies for hot flashes, but there is some support for a daily serving or two of soy protein (it contains plant estrogen), as well as flaxseed. Herbs such as fennel, dong quai, red clover, ginseng, and black cohosh also might be helpful. In addition:

> *Shifty Women...*
> Women working the graveyard shift have a 60 percent higher incidence of breast cancer and a 24 percent increase in pre-term births. Fifty-three percent suffer from altered menstrual cycles. Is the extra pay really worth it?

- Keep your bedroom cool.

- Wear cotton pajamas.

- Use cotton bed sheets.

- Avoid caffeine and alcohol.

Reduce stress throughout the day by managing your time carefully and taking regular power naps and/or meditating.

How is a woman's sleep affected by old age?

As women age, their internal clocks begin to shift, making them tired before their customary bedtime. Mood and movement disorders, chronic pain, health problems, and sleep apnea occur more frequently in postmenopausal women and can cause significant sleep problems. Older people are also more likely to be taking medication that can interfere with sleep. If this is the case, a physician trained in sleep medicine can often suggest less disruptive drugs.

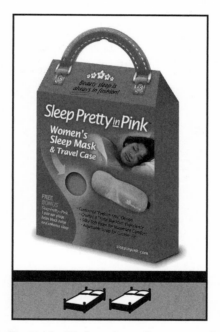

The **Sleep Pretty in Pink** package features a sleep mask, thirty gelcaps containing sleep formula, and pink earplugs to reduce noise by 32 decibels.

Any tips for elderly women trying to log more z's?

It's really important for seniors to get into natural or bright light during the day. This helps set the body's internal clock, or circadian rhythm, so it'll be easier to get to sleep at night. Strive for at least one hour of sunlight per day, and don't keep the lights too dim or low in your house, either. Open those shades or install full-spectrum light bulbs that mimic the natural stuff. Some other tips:

- Set a regular sleep/wake schedule.

- Exercise regularly. Ideally, between 5:00 PM and 7:00 PM.

- Try relaxation techniques.

- Cut out caffeine.

- Don't take naps if you're suffering from insomnia.

- Have regular checkups with your doctor and discuss sleeping problems. If they become a major issue, make an appointment at an accredited sleep-disorder center.

13 Managing Time for Better Sleep

The Real Scoop

How many hours would be in your perfect day? Twenty-five? Thirty? Or would twenty-four be adequate if you could be more alert, efficient, and productive? Since we're stuck with twenty-four, let's make the best of it. Believe it or not, you *can* get everything done—work, friends, spouses, kids, housekeeping, and various other responsibilities—and still leave time for adequate sleep. The secret is twofold: valuing sleep and managing your time. If you get more sleep, you'll be more effective with your time. And if you manage your time, you'll be able to get more sleep. You won't need to slug through the day half-exhausted, and you'll get so much more done. It's a win-win!

What's the effect of chronic sleep deprivation on time management?

Remember, sleep is a necessity, not a luxury. If you're not getting enough sleep regularly, it can and will affect how you use your time. Studies show that one week on six hours or less of sleep per night can bring your brain to the same level as having pulled an all-nighter, and you'll be worse off cognitively than someone who's legally drunk. Needless to say, a sleep pattern like this doesn't lead you to perform at your best. It will make you work slower and focus less, effectively wasting precious time that could be used more productively.

What kind of time wasters are you subject to?

Did you know the more often you switch between tasks, the more time you waste? For example, if you check your e-mail constantly throughout the day, you are continuously disrupting and trying to regain your focus. Imagine writing a budget report when you notice you have

Time Wasters at Work
22% shop online
13% read or create blogs
15% watch videos
18% instant message
10% visit sites like MySpace or Facebook
3% play games

an e-mail. You casually click on your inbox, read and respond to the e-mail, and then click back to your report—what were you writing about again? What was your last thought before you clicked away? The time it takes to answer these questions is precious, especially if you do this several times per day. Fifty-five percent of college students check their e-mail more than three times a day, 37 percent of people with e-mail accounts at work check them constantly, and 54 percent occasionally check their personal e-mail at work.

This last statistic brings us to another time waster—doing things your boss isn't paying you to do! If you shouldn't be getting paid for it, don't do it … This rule will help you save time as well as keep you honest.☺

Why do things always take longer than expected?

People tend to underestimate, rather than overestimate, how long tasks will take. As a result, we often can't finish everything we had planned. Need proof? Estimate how long it will take you to finish this chapter.

"Doc, I know sleep is important, but how can I get enough when I have PTA meetings, little league games, friendships to maintain, and a triathlon to train for?"

Do these concerns sound familiar? Our 24/7 world makes it harder than ever to value sleep. Make a list of your goals. Do you want to be a good father to your children? Do you want to blow last year's sales numbers out of the water and get a raise this year? Do you want to keep improving your running time for a 5K? Then ask yourself what the main things are that consume your time. Do you spend an hour after dinner watching television? Are you spending too long commuting to work because you can't seem to get out the door before rush hour? Are you shopping online or using social networking websites? These thieves take up more of your time than you think. Focus on your goals. Cut everything else out. Make sleep a priority, and you'll likely find that you are a more attentive father, higher performer in the workplace, and better athlete.

What's eating up your time?

The first step to changing how you spend your time is figuring out how you currently spend it. To do this, you'll need to audit yourself for one week. It sounds tedious, but it's necessary! Track how much time you spend doing different activities throughout the day. Ideally, most of these activities will fall into one of your goal categories. The rest can go under the category of "other." Using the data from your time audit, create a pie chart of your goals so you can visualize how you currently distribute your time.

Your Typical Day–Fill it out to see how you're spending your time!	
Time	**Typical Appointments, Tasks, Activities**
8am	
9am	
10am	
11am	
12pm	
1pm	
2pm	
3pm	
4pm	
5pm	
6pm	
7pm	

What changes need to be made?

Now that you know how you spend your time, decide how you *should* be spending your time. This may include talking to supervisors, peers, and family members to determine what your pie chart *should* look like in order to be successful in your role. It may also involve coming up with ways to reduce that pesky little "other" category.

How do you even **begin** *to create an organized schedule?*

This is the biggie for time management—so we'll take it step by step

1. **Where to start.** Use whatever works best for *you* to visually block out your time. This may be buying a planner from the store, creating a calendar on Microsoft Word, using a software tool like Windows Calendar or Google Calendar, or investing in a PDA.

> *What are other people doing?*
>
> "One thing that I do is plan out each of my days. I write down on a post-it note what I'm going to do at each minute of the day. I don't always keep to the schedule, but it helps me to at least have a plan for what I want to accomplish in the day."
> —*Caitlin Royster, a premed student at Cornell University*

2. **Blocking out your time.** Using your new and improved pie chart of how you should be spending your time, block out an appropriate number of hours for each of your goals. For example, a student who wants to spend 20 percent of her fifty-hour school week on homework might designate two-hour blocks each day to "Homework." A well-rounded employee who wants to commit 20 percent of his time each week to his kids might designate two-hour blocks each day to "Being an Involved Parent." This would include taking the kids to soccer practice, playing a game with them, or helping them with their homework. When you're deciding where to place each block, make an Energy Ledger and place high-priority, difficult tasks during the time of day when you are most alert and effective.

> *Avoid the Curse of the Yo-yo Sleep Schedule:*
>
> One part of your schedule that should always be fixed is your sleep. Studies show that people who follow a regular sleep schedule are less sleepy and perform better during the day than people whose sleep schedules jump around.

3. **Create to-do lists within the blocks.** Within your time blocks, create specific to-do lists of everyday things you can do to achieve your block goals. For example, the student mentioned above might list things

such as "calculus assignment," "biology reading," and "English paper" in the "Homework" block. The well-rounded employee might list things such as coaching the soccer team, getting kids ready for school, and spending time with kids at home under the "Being an Involved Parent" block.

4. **Live on a fixed schedule (kind of).** Although some of your blocks can shift around, others may be better at a set time. For example, if you know the gym is always crowded between 5:00 and 8:00 PM or the grocery store has the longest lines around 6:00 PM, fix some parts of your schedule to avoid these inconveniences. Hit the gym during your lunch hour or pick up groceries every Monday before work.

5. **Expect the Unexpected.** Scheduling "contingency time" is probably one of the most important anti-mental-breakdown steps you can take in creating your schedule. Contingency time is a chunk (or chunks) of time in the day where you have absolutely *nothing* scheduled. That way, if you are faced with unexpected obstacles or interruptions, your contingency time can save the day (literally!). Also, remember to schedule tasks for a bit longer than you think they will actually take so you have a buffer zone in case something runs long.

Confessions of a True Time Management Superstar

Tips from Amy Mills, MS, RD, CDN in New York City

I used to run three miles to class at NYU. It took about twenty-five to thirty minutes, the same time as riding the subway. This way, I got my workout done and used that time I would have spent on public transportation getting another thing into my day.

I always grocery shop at off hours, such as during the morning or middle of the day when everyone is at work.

I try to never travel during rush hour except by foot or subway to avoid waiting in traffic.

I make large batches of healthy food on the weekend to eat during the week.

I usually do multiple errands on the same outing and try to group them within the same area.

What if everything won't fit in your schedule?

If this happens, the first thing to do is take a reality check. Ask yourself: Is everything on my list absolutely necessary? Have I taken on too many additional duties? Am I trying to achieve goals in an amount of time that isn't realistic? Am I treating things as more important than they really are? Next, try referring to "TOAD." Use **T**echnology to automate some of your work, **O**utsource whatever you can, see if any tasks can be done in an **A**bbreviated way, and **D**elegate, **D**elegate, **D**elegate! If after this you *still* have a problem getting everything to fit, it may be time to renegotiate your workload. Bring your schedule to your supervisor or advisor and explain that to be successful in your role you may need to lighten your load.

What if you have a procrastination problem?

Unfortunately, there is no easy answer here. The only way to truly overcome procrastination is to face it head on and "power through." The first step is always the hardest, because there never seems to be a right time or right place to start a project. Try thinking of it this way: instead of taking an enormous amount of time to procrastinate on a project (surfing the net, taking care of little projects that could actually wait, making excuses, etc.), use that time to start your project!

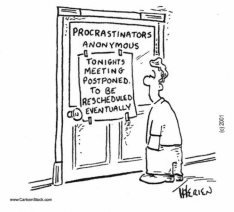

Follow Nike's advice and "Just do it." Motivate yourself with positive thoughts of becoming successful and getting more sleep by sticking to your schedule.

When multitasking is okay.

Save time without compromising quality of work when you combine brainless activities:

- Open your mail while your computer boots up

- Fold laundry while you watch TV

- Unload the dishwasher or clean the kitchen while waiting for coffee to brew

> "Uncluttering your stuff helps you unclutter your mind."
> —*Sandra Block, business owner of "The Clutter Cutter"*

- For students: study flashcards while walking to class (but watch out for potholes and lampposts!)

Fill in the Blanks

What do you do when you have unexpected gaps of five or ten minutes? It's not quite enough time to start a major project, yet it's still too much time to be disregarded as useless. If you find yourself waiting for a meeting to start, sitting on the subway, or waiting for a doctor who fell behind, here are a few things you can do:

- Draw out your schedule for the following week

- Schedule an appointment

- Make a quick phone call

- Do some light reading (it's a good idea to always keep a book or newspaper with you)

- Balance your checkbook

- Meditate—everyone can benefit from five to ten minutes per day of deep breathing and a relaxed mind

When should you respond to e-mails and text messages?

Designate one or two times a day when you will check your e-mail and text messages. Ideally, these will be the times of day when you are most relaxed and have a low level of alertness, such as during your midday dip or at the end of the day when you are still trying to look busy in front of the boss. This will help you reduce the amount of time you spend switching between tasks throughout the day and losing valuable focused time.

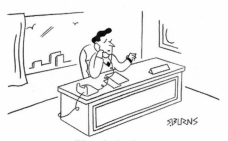

"Hi, good to hear from you. Yes, I'm just back from that time management seminar. Sure, I can talk for a couple of seconds. So, about that meeting tomorr...Oops, time's up. Well, goodbye."

Can you be effective in an unorganized workspace?

Although you may think you can work fine amidst clutter and chaos, chances are you will be more effective if you get organized. How can you do this? First, take everything out of and off of your desk and put it in a big pile. Second, throw away things you don't need. Third, give everything that's left a designated place. Knowing where everything is will help you use your time more efficiently.

Conclusions ...

It *is* possible to get everything done and have enough time for sleep. If you make it a priority to get enough sleep, you will be well-rested, productive, and able to check off your entire to-do list during the day. When it comes to organizing the million and two things you have to do each day, here are some tips: create an Energy Ledger, assess your goals, audit your time, create your ideal schedule, and follow it! If you beat procrastination, multitask effectively, and make use of downtime, you will become a well-rested, time management superstar.

14 Surviving Shift Work

Humans are creatures of the day, so it's no coincidence that most of us work when it's light and sleep at night. But ever since Edison's light bulb hit the market in 1880, we've been trying to cheat the system. We can now keep the world (and ourselves) running 24/7. Indeed, almost 20 percent of US full-time employees have said goodbye to nine-to-five and hello to shift work. And nothing interferes with sleep more. Those who work at night usually aren't able to completely reverse their day and evening cycles. Night-shifters are typically just day-shifters on lots of caffeine.

Scientists suspect that shift work is unhealthy because it disrupts the body's biological clock, or its natural circadian rhythm. For instance, the hormone melatonin, which can suppress tumor development, is normally produced at night. Light depresses melatonin production, so those working in artificial light at night may have lower levels, which scientists speculate can raise cancer risk. Not getting enough sleep also weakens the immune system, making it less able to fight disease.

The Worst Type of Shift Work

There are two basic kinds of shift work, each with its own set of sleep challenges.

About half of shift workers have a regular but unconventional work schedule. A chef might work from 4:00 PM until 2:00 AM, while a security guard is on the job from 10:00 PM until dawn. Because their shifts are consistent, they each have the potential to regularize their sleep cycles. However, they'll have difficulty trying to break that cycle on nights off or holidays.

Then there are those who work rotating or irregular shifts. A hotel clerk might follow a seven-day rotating schedule, sometimes working days and sometimes nights. This is a life of perpetual jetlag (without the exotic destinations). Even worse, an air-traffic controller might work irregular shifts, changing without a pattern. Maintaining any sleep regularity with this schedule is virtually impossible.

Unfortunately, grabbing sleep whenever you can doesn't cut it. Even if the total amount adds up to the recommended nine hours, not following a regular sleep schedule can cause a host of problems.

Why are shift workers at such a disadvantage?

This "biological clock" inside you isn't just a metaphor. Even though you can't hear it ticking, it exists. Its scientific name is the "suprachiasmatic nucleus," or SCN, and it's located in a small but complex region of the brain known as the hypothalamus.

Studies show that this schedule is clearly dictated by light. This body clock adjusts to light by a process called "entrainment," meaning it's slowly pulled into synchronization by its presence, kind of like the moon influences the world's oceans. Anything that promotes entrainment is called a *zeitgeber*, literally a "time-giver" in German. Light is the most important *zeitgeber* to circadian rhythm. Therefore, shift workers are at a tremendous disadvantage when it comes to getting a good night's sleep because their internal clock is at odds with its environment.

How the Boss Should Handle This

If you're a shift worker (or employ shift workers), there are two major factors to take into account when working up your schedule:

1. *Direction of Rotation*

In any given day, your biological clock can accommodate a "phase delay" of two to three hours without too many negative side effects. This basic principle can be applied to the workplace. If possible, make sure that each new shift cycle starts later than the previous one—in other words, move from dayshift to evening shift to nightshift, etc. This progression is the least disruptive to our body clock.

Space/Time Discontinuum

Our twenty-four-hour day doesn't exist in outer space. Humans and other creatures have adapted to earth's rotations around the sun. But astronauts and space workers have to adjust to entirely different schedules.

Scientists working with the Mars Exploration Rover Mission changed their schedules to align with the Martian day. They wore special watches set for days that lasted twenty-four hours, thirty-nine minutes, and thirty-five seconds, and they used our tips to help entrain themselves to new light/dark schedules.

Steve Squyres, PhD, principal investigator for the science instruments on board the Spirit and Opportunity rovers and a Cornell University astronomy professor, said shifting his body clock was tough. "At the start of the Spirit mission, I suddenly had to start working at about 10 pm Pacific time and continue to about 10 am. It was like hopping on a plane and going from New York to Singapore, and it messed me up pretty badly." In retrospect, he concluded that the shift was tolerable as long as earth time didn't "intervene" too much. Adjusting to a permanent schedule, like a consistent night shift, is much easier than constantly changing schedules.

Coming into contact with earth's schedule interfered so much that Squyres tried to avoid it. "I'd schedule family visits once every five weeks, when Mars time was lined up with earth time on the East Coast," he said.

2. *Time between Shift Cycles*

The more time there is between shift cycles, the better. For example, changing shifts every three weeks is much better than changing every week. Likewise, two days off between cycles is better than just one.

Here are some other ideas for the company suggestion box:

- Educate employees about circadian rhythms and sleep strategies.
- Provide breaks, and keep shifts to a reasonable length.
- Provide areas for napping.
- Keep the workspace bright with daylight-spectrum lighting.

Keep in mind, too, that job fatigue is a significant liability concern. If an accident occurs, look at whether scheduling was to blame and if hours of service regulations have been violated.

Employers who respect the biological clock are rewarded with major improvements in productivity—as much as 30 percent with well-designed work schedules.

The Productivity Illusion

In industrialized societies, the push for increased productivity often leads to inadequate sleep for workers. But is there really a linear relationship between hours of work and productivity? As it turns out, there is not. Sleepiness is a confounding variable that is generally ignored.

Fatigued workers cost US employers more than $136 billion per year in lost productivity due to health-related issues. Fatigue and poor health often go together, and this is no coincidence. The study estimated that the prevalence of fatigue in the US workforce is about 38 percent.

7 Steps to Surviving the Night Shift

Since jobs are tough to come by in today's economy, if you or a loved one has to take a job that includes shift work, here are some crucial tips for coping:

1. The most important thing is to stay regular. Go to sleep and wake up at the same time every day, and try to keep to this schedule on nights off and holidays. Simply getting sleep when you can will not cut it.

2. Get an adequate amount of uninterrupted sleep instead of squeezing in a few hours here and there between work and daytime activities.

> **Who's Most at Risk for Fatigue at Work?**
>
> - Women
> - Workers younger than fifty
> - Workers with "high-control" jobs, involving lots of decision-making responsibility

3. Ask friends and family to leave you alone during designated sleep hours. Turn your phone off. Keep your bedroom quiet and comfortable. Invest in thick curtains and carpets to absorb sound.

4. Entrain yourself by using your new knowledge of how light adjusts your body clock. Late afternoon or early evening exposure to bright, daylight-spectrum light, such as Litebook devices (www.litebook.com), can help you reset your clock and keep you awake through the night shift. Keep your work environment equally bright.

5. For the same reasons, be careful not to expose yourself to bright light when you *don't* want to be alert. If you leave work in the morning, wear dark sunglasses on your way home. Make sure your house is dark, even if it's sunny outside. (Bonus: you'll avoid the paparazzi!)

6. Avoid coffee or other caffeinated beverages (and tobacco) toward the end of your shift, and don't have a nightcap

before bed. Alcohol disrupts sleep, even if it initially feels like a tranquilizer.

> **Is Flex Time Healthy?**
>
> Even if your job doesn't involve varying shifts, you might have a lot of flexibility when it comes to when you arrive and leave each day. About 30 percent of the US workforce can vary their hours, according to the Bureau of Labor Statistics. This may seem like a perk, but be careful what you wish for. If you create your own irregular schedule, you're subject to the same complications as shift workers.

7. Sneak away for a twenty-minute power nap during your shift if you feel groggy. It can be dangerous to work while severely sleep-deprived.

Do you have SWSD?

The collection of symptoms that regularly affect shift workers now has an official name: Shift Work Sleep Disorder, or SWSD. The most common symptoms include disrupted sleep, insomnia, irritability, difficulty focusing, headaches, and lack of energy, according to the Washington University Sleep Medicine Center.

SWSD affects about 10 percent of the night- and rotating-shift population. It has been shown to raise the risk of significant behavioral and health-related problems, including sleep-related accidents, ulcers, absenteeism, and depression. Even shift workers who do not suffer from SWSD are likely to be tired more frequently than their day-job counterparts and this, too, can prove dangerous.

How Much Sleep Has My Surgeon Had? (And Other Safety Concerns)

Fatigue is being cited more frequently as a primary cause of major accidents, particularly in hospitals. It's often linked to increases in human error, injuries, and poor performance. Consider:

- Shift workers are forty times more likely than day workers to be involved in accidents—on the job, on the highway, and at home.

- Fatigue is similar to alcohol in its mental effects, impairing concentration, logical reasoning, hand-eye coordination, judgment, and reaction time.

- The probability of serious injury is 43 percent higher during night shifts than day shifts.

    - Some of the greatest workplace catastrophes occurred at night, including the Three Mile Island partial core meltdown in 1979 and the Exxon Valdez oil spill of 1989.

- Work-related fatalities are more than twice as likely to happen during the night shift than the day shift, and the probability of fatalities attributed to human error is also especially high.

- More than half of all shift workers admit to falling asleep on the job at least once a week.

    - A poll of police officers found that 80 percent had fallen asleep once a week while working night shift.

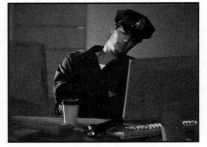

Guilty! More than three-quarters of cops doze on the job.

    - Resident physicians working nights report dozing while taking patient histories and hallucinating during surgical procedures.

What's more?

Shift work takes a serious toll on your health. Shift work is also associated with an increased risk for:

> Sign of the Times: 20 percent of Americans no longer regularly sleep at night.

- Obesity, especially for women.

- Breast and colorectal cancers. The International Agency for Research on Cancer, which is affiliated with the World Health Organization, has classified the aptly named graveyard shift as a "probable cause" of cancer. That puts shift work in the same category as such cancer-causing agents as anabolic steroids, ultraviolet radiation, and diesel-engine exhaust.

- Diabetes.

- Cardiovascular disease.

- Gastrointestinal disease and ulcers.

- Reliance on substances such as alcohol, cigarettes, and coffee to control alertness.

- Mood disorders, depression, and other psychiatric problems.

- Tension, nervousness, and irritability.

- Viral infection—resistance is decreased by 50 percent for shift workers who miss three or more hours of sleep. (Sleep is essential to maintaining the immune system.)

> Lieutenant Chris Estela, infantry officer, works "basically a twenty-four-hour job." He goes to sleep whenever he is told that he should, which varies every night, by anything from one to six hours. "Sometimes you get eight hours of sleep, other times you get zero, so you try to take a nap in the middle of the day, whenever you have downtime," Estela said. He said he has seen people fall asleep while walking or while lying behind a weapon. While "pulling security," he sometimes can't stay awake. "I'll just think that things are happening. I'll slip in and out of consciousness, and I'll keep waking up and thinking that things are real." For Lt. Estela, life without regular sleep is distinctly different from how he remembers life with a nine to five job. "My schedule is really random. And after a while, you kind of just become a zombie. Sometimes you just go through the motions of living."

Less Family Time, Less Sex

When shift workers have time off, they're often so exhausted and so deep in sleep debt that they have trouble fully participating in family and social activities. Shift workers:

- Have difficulty coordinating free time with their children, who have very different schedules.
- Report marital dissatisfaction and problems maintaining sexual relationships with their spouses.
- Must leave evening social events early to go to work or miss many family and social events.

15 Sleep Tips for the Traveler

Have you struggled trying to stay awake in a business meeting seven time zones from home? Have you been excited about a vacation in Paris, only to find yourself dozing off over your Coquilles St. Jacques? The word "travel" originated from the French word "*travailler*" meaning to work hard, but it doesn't have to be so arduous. If you know a few secrets, traveling can be enjoyable, productive, and relaxing rather than stressful and exhausting. Here's your itinerary:

Air Travel: Are you time-zoned out?

Jetlag is the air traveler's worst nightmare. It occurs when you cross multiple time zones (usually three or more) in a short period. Travel was slower before airplanes, and it often took several days to reach a destination. By the time you arrived by train, car, or ship, your body had already adjusted to the shift. Now we're able to jet over multiple zones in a matter of hours, but our internal biological clocks can't acclimate that fast, and we feel out of synch. The effects are most pronounced when flying east or west.

What are the main symptoms of jetlag?

- *Daytime sleepiness*

  Ninety percent of all travelers crossing multiple time zones are plagued by daytime drowsiness. This can last for a week or more.

- *Insomnia*

  The jetlagged feel restless and can't get to sleep or stay asleep, waking up either too early or too late depending on their direction of travel.

- *Poor concentration*

  This is especially disruptive for those traveling on business. It can take several days to fully recover and regain mental alertness. Symptoms include foggy memory, inattentiveness, lack of focus, and temporary amnesia.

- *Slower reaction times*

  Two-thirds of travelers have slower response times and poor visual focus. Night vision and peripheral vision also decline. This can make any task that requires full alertness extremely dangerous, such as driving (or diving, see sidebar).

Jetting Blues

A survey of international flight attendants found that while they were "accustomed" to long-haul travel, 90 percent suffered from fatigue the first five days after arrival, 94 percent experienced a lack of energy and motivation, 93 percent reported fragmented sleep, and 70 percent had ear, nose, or throat problems.

Diver Greg Louganis struck his head on the ten-meter platform during the 1979 Olympic Trials and was unconscious for twenty minutes. His acrobatic skills and precision timing had been affected by jetlag.

Aloha Air

Senator Hiram Fong retired because the 9,116-mile flight between his home in Hawaii and his office in Washington DC was too debilitating. He did the trip eighteen times per year and suffered from chronic jetlag.

- *Indigestion/gastrointestinal problems*
  Jetlag affects your stomach, too. Half of all travelers experience hunger pangs, diarrhea, constipation, indigestion, or heartburn. It also can worsen ulcers. Not fun, especially when you're far from home.

> **Death by Jetlag**
>
> Sarah Krasnoff, seventy-four, kidnapped her fourteen-year-old grandson after losing a custody dispute. Realizing that they wouldn't be subject to the law if they continued to fly, they jetted back and forth between New York and Amsterdam 160 times. During the course of these flights, they watched twenty-two different movies, seven times each. After repeatedly turning their watches forward six hours and then back six hours, Krasnoff could no longer handle the constant time changes. She collapsed and died from what was determined by doctors as terminal jetlag, ending her "fugitive enterprise."

Does it matter how many time zones I'm crossing?

Yes, depending on your sensitivity to time change, jetlag starts becoming apparent after you cross three time zones. After that, it usually takes about one day to recover from each zone crossed.

However, if you were to fly around the world, passing through each of the twenty-four time zones and returning to the place where you started, you wouldn't suffer any jetlag and your biological clock would be unaltered. But you would be one tired puppy!

Does the direction of flight affect the severity of jetlag?

Yes. Eastbound flights or those going counter to the direction of the sun cause more severe jetlag than westbound ones. It can take up to 50 percent longer to recover from flying east than flying west. That's because you're shortening the day. Thus, to stay on schedule when flying from Los Angeles to New York, you must go to bed earlier than you would back home. Most times, though, you'll have difficulty falling asleep and getting up the next morning. When flying west, the day is lengthened. As a result, you'll tend to fall asleep and wake up earlier.

If you're traveling one or two time zones from home for just a few days, it's easier to maintain your usual schedule, arranging meetings or activities for when you're normally most alert.

Does my age or personality affect the severity of jetlag?

Children under age three seem to be unaffected by jetlag, but the older you get the more it impacts your body and mind. People over age sixty often take weeks to recover from crossing more than six time zones, and although flying east is usually more detrimental, senior citizens have more difficulty traveling westward. Interestingly, outgoing, gregarious, and social people, as well as people who tend to be more flexible, find it easier to adjust to time-zone change than reserved, shy, and tranquil folks.

What can I do to minimize or prevent jetlag?

1. Pre-flight

- *Adjust your biological clock.* Four or five days before a major eastbound trip (say, from New York to London), start eating dinner and going to bed one hour earlier each night. If heading west, stay up and get up later.

- *Avoid early-morning departures.* You'll be so worried that you'll miss your flight that you'll toss and turn all night. Plus, you'll probably be up late packing, which will reduce total sleep time.

- *Arrive at your destination in time for a full night's sleep.* Don't make the mistake of thinking you'll sleep on the plane, freshen up in the washroom, and then head right to your meeting. Instead, arrive a day early and get some rest. If the meeting is important enough to fly to, then it's important enough for you to be in top form.

- *Avoid red-eye flights.* Although you'll save some time and a night in a hotel, the cost of losing sleep is usually even greater. In terms of mood, health, and performance, you won't be the same for days afterward.

- *Pre-select a comfortable seat.* Choose one that reclines (those in emergency rows don't) and one that offers a little extra legroom (any on the aisle). Steer clear of bathrooms and galleys, which have a lot of traffic, or bulkhead seats where infants are often placed. Also consider which side of the plane the sun will be on and sit opposite it.

- *Allow plenty of time.* Arriving at the airport early makes things less stressful, plus it betters your chances for an upgrade.

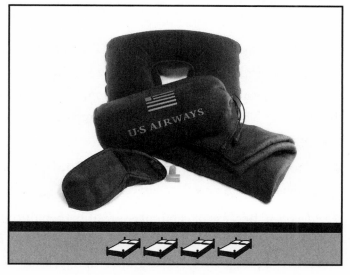

The *US Airways Power-Nap Sack™* can be purchased in flight and contains all of your airtime napping essentials.

- *Spread out.* At the gate, ask the boarding agent if there are any empty rows—three vacant seats make a quasi-bed.

- *Pack a "sleeping bag."* No, not the camping sort, but rather a stash of feel-good items that will keep you comfortable. Include an eye mask, earplugs, slipper socks, gum (for equalizing ear pressure on takeoff and landing), moisturizer, lip balm, and a nasal decongestant. Wear loose-fitting clothes and dress in layers for warmth and comfort.

- *Don't leave trip preparations until the last minute.* Be well rested, not exhausted, when you start your journey.

2. In-flight

- *Snag a pillow and blanket as soon as you board.* Many airlines no longer carry enough for everyone.

- *As soon as you're seated, change your watch to "destination time."* Forget the airline's schedule. Even though it's still daytime outside the plane, if it's nighttime at your destination, forget the movie and meals, tell the cabin crew you do not wish to be disturbed, and get some sleep.

- *Drink lots of water and juice to counter dehydration.* The humidity in airplane cabins is so low that it dehydrates your body without you realizing it. Dehydration, which depresses the ability of blood to carry oxygen, can retard the process of re-synchronizing your biological clock.

- *Avoid stimulants.* Caffeine and nicotine disturb sleep and delay adjustment to new time zones.

- *Avoid alcohol.* Because of cabin pressure at higher altitudes, two drinks in the air are as potent as three drinks on the ground. Despite how tempting that may sound, don't compound the effects of jetlag with a hangover.

It's the end of the world ... (and I feel fine). Many people turn to prescription sleeping pills to help them relax on planes. But use them judiciously so you're not groggy upon arrival. Be aware that some medications, such as Ambien, have been linked to bizarre sleepwalking incidents, including air rage. Guitarist Peter Buck (whose band is ironically named REM) was eventually cleared of assault and drunkenness charges stemming from his destructive rampage aboard a British Airways flight. He claimed that taking Ambien—combined with several glasses of wine—caused "non-insane automatism," which rendered him unable to control his actions.

- *Watch what you eat.* Having a couple of burritos or a pepperoni pizza before boarding will make it even more challenging to get comfortable. It's better to pack food so you can eat on your own schedule.

- *Use noise-canceling headphones.* These reduce fatigue from engine and passenger noise.

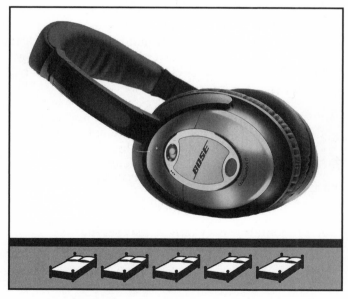

Bose QuietComfort® 15 Acoustic Noise Cancelling® headphones reduce travel fatigue significantly by masking engine roar and annoying cabin sounds.

Image of QuietComfort® 15 Headphones used with permission from Bose Corporation.

- *Remove contact lenses.* This will avoid dryness, irritation, and seeing how much room everyone in business class has.

- *Cover yourself with a blanket.* This will ensure you're comfortable as body temperature drops from inactivity and sleep.

- *Use a light-generating gadget to help reset your biological clock.* You can simulate daytime during a night flight with a battery-operated, artificial-light gadget such as the Litebook (www.litebook.com). Don't worry; these won't flood the entire cabin. They can be set to shine obliquely and are best used for reading when you wake up and it's already morning at your destination.

- *If necessary, consider an antihistamine to induce sleep.* Tylenol PM or Benadryl are effective. However, because adults may build a tolerance to these drugs, they are often more useful with children.

> **Melatonin & Jetlag:** Some travelers take melatonin, the hormone that regulates our wake/sleep cycles, in order to reduce jetlag. The problem in America is that melatonin is considered a supplement and is not regulated by the FDA. So we don't know its purity or its long-term effects. Although it's less addictive than prescription drugs, inappropriate dosages can produce mood-altering side-effects. The bottom line is: forget the melatonin.

- *Take a hike.* Stroll down the aisle periodically to improve blood circulation. When muscles become tense from immobility, heavy fatigue may set in.

Simple In-Flight Stretching Program: These easy exercises can be done in your seat to help you stay limber and also build energy prior to arrival. If you're worried about what the other people in your row will think, invite them to join you.

- **Deep breathing**—(6 repetitions) Breathe deeply through your nose and exhale slowly through your mouth. This helps disperse fresh oxygen throughout the body, which helps adjust your biological clock.

- **Arm and torso stretches**—(6 repetitions) Raise one arm at a time as if you were trying to pick an apple. You should feel a stretch down the side of your torso. Hold for one minute on each side. (Hopefully the flight attendant will not think you're signaling for another round.)

- **Neck rotations**—(6 repetitions) From the looking-straight-ahead position, slowly turn your head to the left and hold. Then do the same to the right.

- **Head nods**—(6 repetitions) To stretch the back of your neck, slowly drop your chin to your chest and hold for a few seconds. Then gently tilt your head back to stretch the front of your neck.

- **Shoulder rolls**—(6 repetitions) Slowly move both of your shoulders forward in large circles and then switch direction.

- **Wrist rotations**—(10 repetitions) Spread your fingers in an open-hand position. Rotate your wrists clockwise, then counter-clockwise.

- **Ankle circles**—(10 repetitions) Rotate your feet in large circles, first in one direction and then the other.

- **Knee lifts**—(10 repetitions) Bring your right knee to your left elbow, and then your left knee to your right elbow to stimulate blood flow.

- **Arm jogs**—(2 minutes) Swing your arms back and forth continuously as if you were jogging. In two minutes you'll cover approximately twenty-three air miles—almost an entire marathon!

- **Seat lifts**—(10 repetitions) Without using your hands, get up from your seat and then sit back down to stimulate circulation.

- **Stomach stretches**—(10 repetitions) Pull in your gut and then bend forward. While bent over, relax stomach muscles and sit up. Don't expect to have abs by the time you get to Austin, though.

3. Post-flight

- *If you flew east* … and it's morning at your destination but still the middle of the night in your head, don't go to sleep. Even though you're exhausted, it's far better to push through the day and fall into bed early that evening. Get out in the sun as soon as possible. Daylight is a powerful stimulant for regulating your biological clock. Staying indoors actually worsens jetlag.

- *If you flew west ...* and it's already evening according to your biological clock, spend time outdoors in the afternoon sun. The light will help you feel fresher and adjust your internal clock.

- *Check into a sleep-friendly hotel ...* That's right. Hotels are going way beyond the pillow mint to help you sleep better.

Check in Here (and Really Check Out)

- *Westin Hotels* were the first major chain to install high-end mattresses, "Heavenly Beds," in their hotel rooms.

- *The Hotel Gabriel Paris Marais* claims they are the world's best detox hotel. They outfit rooms with "night core," a system that uses light and sound to lull you to sleep.

- *The Sheraton* offers an exercise and nutrition program which includes an energy-rich menu with items that help travelers minimize the effects of jetlag.

- *Jumeriah and Conrad Hotels* offer "pillow menus" from which guests can choose what they want to lay their heads on.

---

4. When you check in ...

- *Request an out-of-the-way room.* Limit noise by reserving a room on an upper floor and away from elevators, stairways, vending or ice machines, hospitality rooms, and, of course, the honeymoon suite. If that's not possible, use earplugs or turn the air-conditioner fan on high to mask noise.

- *Ask for a room with an eastern or southern exposure for more morning sun.* If you've traveled from the west this will make it easier to become alert in the morning. (If you're south of the equator, get a room with an eastern or northern exposure.)

- *Pull the drapes at night to block city light and reduce noise.* Pack clothespins to hold them closed in case they don't overlap.

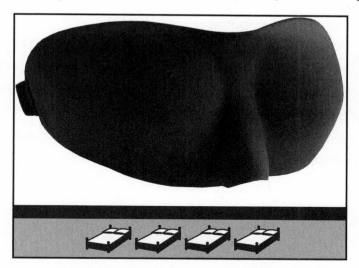

The **Sweet Dreams Contoured Sleep Mask** is made of lightweight foam surrounded by polyester for a comfortable experience.

- *Keep the room at 65 degrees.* Check the thermostat when you arrive and call management if there's a problem adjusting it.

- *Request extra pillows or blankets when you check in.* Maid service is sometimes hard to come by late at night. If you have a favorite pillow and some extra space in your luggage, bring it.

- *Get some exercise.* If you need to stay up, even a brisk walk after a long flight will raise endorphin levels. This will reduce stiffness and pain, relax your muscles, and suppress drowsiness.

- *Pack a nightlight so you can navigate the room.* This will make you feel more secure, and it'll keep you from flicking on the bright, sleep-disrupting overhead if you need to go to the bathroom in the wee hours of the morning.

- *Bolt the door and hang out the "Do not disturb" sign.* This promotes safety and keeps confused guests from trying to get into your room.

- *Set the alarm and request a wake-up call.* This provides double insurance that you won't oversleep, which eases worry if you have an early appointment. While you're at it, ask the operator to hold all calls until morning.

- *Leave it for Day 2.* If you have important business or are competing in sports and have traveled across five time zones, just relax on the day of arrival. Otherwise, mistakes will be made, negotiations will suffer, and all that training will be wasted.

Car Travel: Drowsy driving is drunk driving

Many drivers insist they can tell when they're about to fall asleep, but research shows otherwise. Most drivers who nod off do so without knowing it. Sleep expert Dr. William C. Dement says many people experience "microsleeps" or "uncontrollable and unpredictable bouts of sleep that happen faster than a seizure." We may fall asleep only for a few seconds, but, behind the wheel of car, a lot of damage can be done in that instant.

> "Two days before our wedding, my fiancé was killed by a drowsy driver. Wedding plans changed to funeral plans, groomsmen became pall-bearers, and instead of walking down the aisle in white, I wore black. It was all so pointless."
> —*Young widow Amy Huther*

Who is most susceptible to drowsy driving?

Teens, without a doubt. They're learning to drive, experimenting with drinking, and are the most sleep-deprived members of society. The peak hours for drowsy driving in this group are midnight to 6:00 AM (and,

incidentally, when most drowsy-driving accidents occur), which is why some states have instituted curfews. Stimulation from socializing and partying generally masks sleepiness until you get in the car and start heading home.

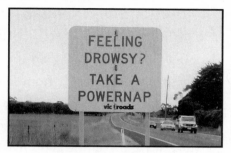

The second largest risk group is people over age sixty-five. The elderly most often fall asleep

Get Pulled Over: A fifteen- to twenty-minute nap will refresh but only supply about thirty more minutes of alert driving time.

during midday hours. And night workers can doze off early in the morning when driving home after the ironically named graveyard shift.

How do I know if I'm driving drowsy?

Here are the warning signs, according to the American Automobile Association. Although they may seem obvious, it's amazing how many people don't recognize or heed them:

- Uncontrollable yawning
- Heavy eyelids
- Loss of focus
- Drooping head
- Wandering thoughts
- Memory loss of how you got from place to place

- Drifting lanes, tailgating, and missing traffic signals

- Continually jerking the car back into the lane or drifting off of the road

How can I stay awake if I feel myself getting drowsy?

Opening windows, turning on the air conditioning, or cranking the radio will *not* prevent you from falling asleep at the wheel if you're sleep-deprived. If you experience any of the symptoms of drowsy driving outlined earlier, pull over immediately to a safe area, lock your doors, and take a nap. Well-lit and busy rest areas are generally the most secure, or park in an open gas station or convenience store lot. A fifteen- to twenty-minute power nap will only supply about thirty more minutes of driving time, though. Get some caffeinated coffee or cola and take a brief brisk walk before resuming your trip.

Remember that if you've experienced one or more of the warning signs, you're driving impaired and are endangering yourself and others.

So what can I do to stay safe during a long road trip?

- *Start well rested.* Driving requires total mental and physical alertness. So get adequate sleep the week before and especially the night before you leave.

- *Don't rely on Joe.* If you feel you need caffeinated drinks or over-the-counter medications to stay awake, you're probably too tired to drive. Although caffeine will give you a short burst of energy, it's not a replacement for real rest and alertness.

- *Keep it under ten.* Don't drive for more than ten hours, which is the legal limit for operators of commercial vehicles.

- *Stay on schedule.* Try to drive during the times of day when you're normally most alert.

- *Avoid driving through the night.* Your body craves sleep after dark. You're programmed that way, so don't fight it. The glare of oncoming lights also increases the danger of highway hypnosis.

- *Don't put yourself in a time bind.* Plan for congestion, bad weather, and unpredictable delays by leaving a bit early. Stress is fatiguing.

- *If possible, don't drive alone.* Conversation and sharing the driving load relieves tiredness and monotony.

- *Be slightly uncomfortable.* Adjust the car temperature and environment so it's not too pleasant. Keep the temperature cool and avoid listening to soft, sleep-inducing music.

- *Don't use cruise control.* Keep your body and brain involved in the driving process.

- *Sit up tall.* Slouching can induce fatigue. Drive with your head up and shoulders back. (Setting the rearview mirror a little higher encourages this.) Legs should be flexed at about a 45-degree angle.

- *Take frequent breaks.* Stop and get out of the car at least once every two hours, or every one hundred miles. Eat a light, protein-rich snack to facilitate alertness. Chewing gum also helps keep you sharp.

- *Exercise during your breaks.* Move your body briskly to increase heart rate and boost alertness.

- *Monitor your medications.* Avoid driving if you have used drugs that induce drowsiness.

- *Do not consume alcohol.* Even one drink, if you're tired, can severely impair your ability to drive.

- *Move those eyeballs.* Instead of staring straight ahead, scan your mirrors and the road, blinking frequently and naturally.

- *Book the roadside Ritz.* If you're driving for consecutive days, make sure you get a good sleep the nights in between.

- *Don't risk it.* If you suspect you may have a sleep disorder, see your doctor. If he's particularly well-to-do, ask if he can recommend a good chauffeur.

Exceeding the Sleep Limit:

Joshua was the youngest of my three children. He was such a happy-go-lucky kid, with a kind heart and a loving, sensitive personality. On March 14, 2004, he was on his way to Montana with his dad when they were hit head-on by a nineteen-year-old National Guardsman who had been up for fifty-six straight hours of duty. He fell asleep at the wheel with his cruise control set at seventy mph. A witness stated that my husband swerved to avoid the crash, but there was nothing he could do. Joshua and his father were killed immediately, and myself and our other two children didn't have a chance to say goodbye. The man who hit them did not receive any type of punishment, nor was he even charged. The police chief told me, "I have no intentions of filing charges on that young man; he was on his way home from military training."
—*Submitted by Tawna Andrews*

---

16 Sleep, Exercise, and the Athlete

Exercise is an integral part of a healthy person's daily routine. It improves mood and general health, and it increases your lifespan. Moreover, when you exercise on a regular basis, you'll find it easier to fall asleep and maintain sleep. What you might not know is that adequate sleep can *dramatically* improve your athletic ability, whether you're training for next year's Boston Marathon or just hoping to beat your kids at Wii boxing. And it doesn't require more training, high-tech equipment, or (for aging folks) any titanium knee replacements. What you're about to learn will bring new meaning to the term "in the zone."

> "I've been training for triathlons the past six years, and I usually sleep four to five hours per night. After attending one of Dr. Maas' presentations, I did an experiment. I added one extra hour of sleep every night from that Monday through Sunday, when I had a four-mile race. Without working any harder, I crushed my personal record by almost a minute—a significant improvement. All attributable to sleep."
> —*David Brinker, MD*

Swap the Sominex for Reeboks:

People who work out regularly have a more defined circadian rhythm; when they're alert, they're more alert than their sedentary counterparts, and at bedtime they're drowsier than those who aren't active. And if you think you don't have enough time to exercise, think of all the time you're wasting every night tossing and turning in bed.

Is there scientific proof that adequate sleep improves athletic performance?

Many studies have found undeniable connections between sleep and athletic performance. Well-rested subjects are typically 20 percent quicker at performing physical tasks than those who lack adequate rest. Sleep plays a major role in strengthening the bonds between brain cells involved in muscle memory, thus sharpening focus, reducing reaction time, and even enhancing energy, attitude, and motivation.

Is any one stage of sleep more essential than another for enhancing athletic performance?

While REM sleep often takes center stage, your athletic excellence is dependent on several actors in the theater of the night. Here's why:

REM sleep promotes learning. After a day of learning new techniques, skills, and strategies, there is a significant increase in brain activity during REM sleep. This stage helps strengthen neural connections created during practice. So, after you take a tennis lesson, getting an adequate amount of REM sleep will allow those new skills to become part of your long-term "muscle memory." In your next match, you'll be able to apply those skills automatically. But REM sleep alone isn't enough to bring optimal results.

Slow–wave sleep (SWS) promotes muscle growth and recovery. This type of sleep, found predominantly in Stages 3 and 4, is essential for athletes because it's when the body produces human growth hormone (HGH).

This process creates the proteins necessary for muscle development and recovery. Weight training and workouts can't make you stronger without this vital hormone.

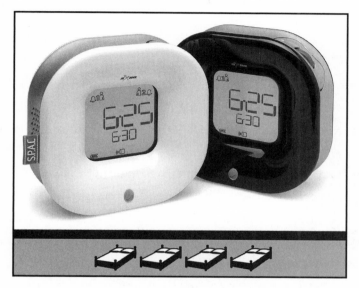

aXbo is the world's first sleep-phase alarm clock. It wakes you up while you are in a light sleep phase so that you maximize alertness when you wake up. And it will go off early enough so that you're not late for work!

Stage 2 "sleep spindles" promote muscle memory. Stage 2 sleep, which occurs predominantly during the last quarter of a good, eight-hour night's sleep, is marked by the formation of "sleep spindles." These bursts of brain activity represent a cascade of calcium into the motor cortex and the pyramidal tract—areas of the brain associated with muscle memory and control. This increase in calcium can only be triggered by sleep, not calcium supplements. This heightened calcium concentration turns on specific enzymes that create lasting muscle memories for step-by-step sequences, such as the components of a golf swing. If you had to think through everything you must do in the 1.5 seconds between drawing a driver back and striking the ball, you'd never be in the fairway. Instead,

Stage 2 (and REM) sleep enables us to memorize that sequence for quick, subconscious recall. Since the majority of these spindles form between the sixth and eighth hour of rest, if you're sleep-deprived you're missing the opportunity to be a better athlete.

When is the best time to train or compete?

Your core body temperature, which is linked to your circadian rhythm, fluctuates naturally throughout the day. Synchronizing workouts and competitive events with the peaks in these temperature cycles is one secret to enhancing performance.

The body's need for sleep and its circadian rhythm work in tandem throughout each twenty-four-hour period, creating peaks and troughs in alertness. These same forces dictate the best times for training and competing. Here's how to take advantage of your natural peaks and troughs in alertness:

Avoid strenuous morning exercise: Body temperature is lowest as we're waking up, usually between 7:00 AM and 10:00 AM. It takes several hours after awakening for our bodies to build back up to an optimum temperature for alertness. Exercising during this adjustment period increases core temperature too quickly and disrupts this process, causing overheating and exhaustion.

In addition, fluid accumulates between the discs in our spinal cord during the night. Exercising immediately after awakening without stretching for at least thirty minutes makes us more prone to injury (lower back pain and a risk of herniating a disk) because this fluid doesn't have time to dissipate.

A late-afternoon workout is ideal: The optimal time for exercise is between 5:00 PM and 7:00 PM because the body is neither trying to accumulate heat nor disperse it. In this window, the body's natural cooling methods respond quickest to the increase in body temperature from exercising, allowing you to avoid overheating and work out longer and harder with less perceived effort. This window is also past the usual midday dip in alertness (typically between 2:00 PM and 4:00 PM) when core body temperature naturally drops and reaction time slows.

Say no to nighttime workouts: Body temperature is at its highest between 9:00 PM and midnight, prompting the drowsiness that eventually tucks you in. However, in order to allow for sleep, some of this heat needs to be shed. That's why exercising in the evening is counterproductive: your body is trying to cool down, but late-night exercise warms you up for hours afterwards. As a general rule, never exercise within three hours of bedtime, or you won't be able to fall asleep. An exception to the rule: satisfying sex, which can promote deep sleep.

Why do I feel so tired and out of breath some days when I'm exercising?

It's probably because you didn't get enough sleep the previous night. Studies show that when you're sleep-deprived and exercising intensely, you suffer an 8 percent decline in VO_2 max (the maximum volume of oxygen your body can process), a 14 percent reduction in anaerobic power (the body's ability to function without oxygen), and a significant increase in heart rate and lactic acid (the chemical that makes muscles sore). So when you're in this state, your heart is beating unnecessarily hard and your muscles are working against themselves. Lack of sleep makes you an inefficient athlete.

Can't I sneak by on six hours or less of sleep per night?

You may be able to get by, but you won't excel. Getting reduced sleep or sleep that is of poor quality has the same negative effects on performance as not sleeping at all. Losing sleep slows the process of glucose metabolism, or the conversion of sugar into muscle fuel. Studies have shown this process slows by nearly 40 percent in as little as one week. For endurance athletes, such as runners and cyclists, this means that working muscles aren't receiving adequate energy. Thus, the sensation of "hitting the wall" or "bonking" occurs 20 percent sooner than in well-rested athletes. That's an enormous margin. Imagine a well-rested runner who's usually exhausted at the finish of a one-mile race. Now take the same runner at the same speed and deprive him of sleep; he'll be used up with three-quarters of a lap to go.

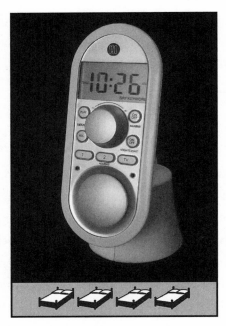

The Accenda Sunshine is a voice-activated talking alarm clock that will also record memos which will be announced at the designated time. It is also voice activated so it can work hands free and you can set your alarm clock as you're falling asleep without having to move a muscle, other than your mouth!

Can energy drinks or foods boost performance enough to make up for poor sleep?

Sorry, but you can't buy your way out of sleep loss. Store shelves are packed with products that claim to postpone exhaustion. While their sugar and caffeine content can deliver a short-term boost, they won't reverse the negative effects of chronic sleep loss. Save your money—go to sleep.

> *Feeling sluggish on the track or in the office?* Use exercise as a tool to get through those times when lack of sleep is turning your mind and muscles into molasses. One of the best ways to boost alertness at any time of day, whether you're an athlete or not, is to exercise. Just five minutes of exercise is incredibly effective in reducing drowsiness. So if you're studying and having a hard time staying awake, go for a brisk five-minute walk. If you're about to attend a budget meeting and you're worried about falling asleep on the CEO, do some jumping jacks or push-ups in your office beforehand or during the break.

Is it true that muscular strength isn't affected by sleep loss?

Muscle strength is the facet of athletic performance that's most resistant to sleep loss. Even after a sleepless night, weightlifters can usually heft just as much iron and sprinters can run just as fast in a single, all-out burst of energy. However, even muscle strength shows marked deterioration after two nights of inadequate rest. Therefore, count back two nights before your event and make that your key night of sleep. Even if your schedule can't accommodate eight to ten hours on a regular basis, at least set that night apart for a long and restful sleep.

So if my muscle strength is unaffected, what's the big deal?

Muscle strength alone does not make an athlete. Reaction time, attitude, precision, and immunity are just a few of the other essential elements, all of which are significantly enhanced by sleep. Here's a rundown on why you're run down after poor sleep:

Reaction time slows. Although it's only by a few fractions of a second, if you're a fan of the Olympics you know that's often the difference between the podium and a long trip home. It was a margin of only

0.08 seconds that won the gold medal for Jason Lezak and the US 4x100-meter free relay team at the 2008 Beijing Games. It was just 0.01 seconds that made the difference in Michael Phelps' victory in the 100-meter butterfly.

Positive attitudes turn sour. In one study, swimmers who slept for four hours the previous night were tested for mood. They showed far more irritability and loss of enthusiasm than their well-rested peers. You know what they say: attitude is everything.

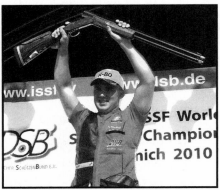

This guy is a straight shooter...
"I was fortunate to win the Gold Medal at the 2010 World International Shooting Championship in Munich, Germany. I placed 2nd at the United States National Championship, set two USA Junior National Records, won the USA Junior National Championship and the USA Junior Olympic Championship. I have continued to make your research, findings and suggestions part of my training. For each event, I made it a primary focus to get 9 hours of sleep or more."

Jon Michael McGrath II
UNITED STATES SHOTGUN TEAM

Precision plummets. Research shows that a full night's sleep will increase the accuracy of your movements. Does your baseline jumper keep falling short? Are you consistently swinging just under fastballs? Then spending a little less time practicing and a little more time sleeping could actually raise both your shooting and batting averages. A study of women varsity tennis players at Stanford showed that more sleep can significantly improve athletic performance. Extending their sleep to ten hours each night was associated with faster sprinting drills and increased hitting accuracy. Their daytime sleepiness and fatigue also decreased, and their vigor improved. The results are consistent with similar studies previously conducted with Stanford athletes in other sports.

Immunity suffers. Losing sleep depresses your immune system. You need rest to ensure you're healthy for competition. Plus, when you train you're literally destroying microscopic bits of muscle. These "micro-tears" require time to repair, helping the muscle grow thicker and stronger in response to the added stress. Think of sleep as protection against muscle deterioration.

Do twice-daily workouts lead to success or burnout?

Traditionally, many coaches have considered two daily workouts to be essential for athletic success. But if one of these sessions is in the early morning, it's probably doing more harm than good. Early-morning training robs athletes of valuable sleep and makes them prone to injury and illness. It's much better to have well-rested athletes practice hard in the 5:00 PM to 7:00 PM time period. There are countless case histories of athletes and athletic teams that have dropped early-morning practices and found greater success in competition. This holds true for sports as diverse as basketball, football, wrestling, lacrosse, swimming, and figure skating.

> *What happens when you cut early-morning practice?*
> —Cornell University's men's basketball team wins the Ivy League title and makes the NCAA tournament Sweet Sixteen for the first time.
> —New York Jets improve their record from 4-12 to 9-7 in one season.
> —US figure skater Sarah Hughes wins the Olympic gold medal.

Can the quality of my sleep tell me anything about how I'm training?

How you're sleeping won't tell you a lot about the appropriateness of a particular type of conditioning, but it can tell you something about the amount of training you're doing. If you're consistently working out very hard, not seeing any performance gains, and finding it difficult to sleep, you may be suffering from Overtraining Syndrome (OTS). In fact, sleep disturbances and mood changes are major indicators of this condition. Since the body thrives on balance, always try to counter strenuous exercise with the appropriate amount of rest.

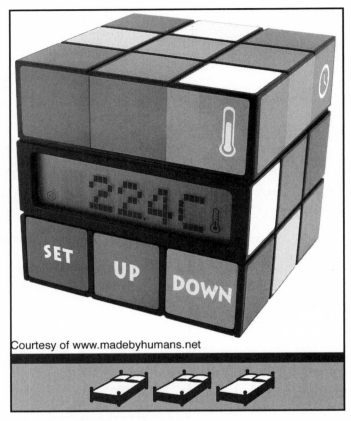

Courtesy of www.madebyhumans.net

The **Rubiks Cube Clock** is a "just for fun" gadget that can be rotated to adjust what you want it to display: time, temperature, date, or alarm.

How does air travel affect athletic performance?

Because regular exercisers have such well-synchronized circadian rhythms, anything that disrupts the body's natural cycle, such as a cross-country flight, can be devastating. Many athletes traveling across multiple time zones report a significant increase in daytime drowsiness even when they can stick to their normal sleep schedule upon arrival.

So it looks like the requisite 8 to 9.25 hours of nighttime rest won't cut it. You may need to add extra nighttime sleep and naps to compensate. And remember, it takes approximately one day to adjust to a new sleep/wake schedule per time zone crossed.

> *Participating in a competition several time zones away?* Arrive at your destination a couple of days prior to the event. You must acclimate yourself to the foreign conditions and be well rested in order to perform at an optimum level. If you're only traveling across one or two time zones, consider keeping your watch set to home time and eating and sleeping accordingly. Just don't miss your start!

Do naps enhance performance?

Naps are just as beneficial for athletes as they are for everyone else. Taking a twenty-minute nap can lower your heart rate, improve your reaction time, and increase your explosive power. However, be sure to nap no longer than twenty minutes, especially prior to an afternoon or evening event, or else you'll wake up groggy and your movements will be lethargic.

> *Snooze for Skills:* The night after learning a new skill or technique in your sport, the time spent in Stage 2 sleep and the number of sleep spindles increase. This is the driving factor behind a decrease in the number of errors in completing the new task after a full night's rest.

How much sleep is optimal for an athlete?

Athletes need more rest and recovery time than sedentary people because of all the additional muscle fatigue and mental exhaustion. The traditional 8 to 9.25 hours of sleep is adequate for an athlete, but to truly achieve peak performance, extra rest time is needed. Indeed, sleep is so important that it probably deserves a slot on training schedules. If you're a promising high-school quarterback with dreams of a scholarship, or a weekend warrior with a summer triathlon goal, then sleep may be worth prioritizing. Experiment with different amounts to see how it affects your performance and attitude. Who knows? You might just turn yourself into a superstar (at least in the eyes of those who really love you)!

PART Five

An Up-to-Date Look at Sleep Disorders and Their Treatment

17
Understanding and Treating the Most Common Sleep Disorders

We've done our best to make you comfortable, tuck you in, and ensure that you'll get a good night's sleep. But some of you will still end up tossing and turning. If this is your situation, if none of the advice we've given so far has worked, you're probably being stalked by the ultimate bogeyman: a sleep disorder.

To ascertain if this is the case, ask yourself these questions:

- Do you repeatedly have difficulty falling asleep, staying asleep, or waking up too early?

- Do you feel drowsy during the day?

- Do you experience creepy-crawly sensations in your legs when you lie down that can only be alleviated by moving around?

- Do you suddenly lose muscle control and sometimes even collapse when experiencing strong emotion such as laughter or shock?

- Have you ever awakened in a strange place and wondered how you got there?

- Did you ever awaken with food in your bed and wonder how it got there?

- Has your bed partner ever told you that you tried to make love while asleep?

Believe it or not, these are all characteristics of some of the eighty-nine different, diagnosable sleep disorders. In this chapter, we'll review the most common (and bizarre) while providing some advice and solutions. So read on if you need answers on why you're so tired during the day or what the heck that pork chop was doing under your pillow.

INSOMNIA

Why, if I've done everything you've recommended, am I still having difficulty falling asleep, staying asleep, or waking up too early?

You probably have insomnia. This sleep disorder can have many causes, ranging from physical (hormonal fluctuations or pain) to psychological (anxiety or depression) to situational (noise or jetlag). Just being older or female can predispose you to it.

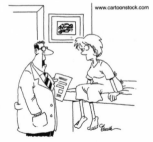

"It's nothing to lose any sleep over. You just have insomnia."

Insomnia has far-reaching effects on health, mood, concentration, response time, general performance, and overall quality of life. Because of this, it's important to seek medical and/or behavioral treatment to remedy it.

Are there different types of insomnia?

Yes, there are many. *Transient insomnia* is a sleep disturbance that generally lasts for three weeks or fewer. *Intermittent insomnia* is recurring transient insomnia. *Chronic insomnia* is persistent, long-lasting sleep loss, occurring on most nights.

These three main types are further subdivided into *sleep-onset insomnia* (trouble falling asleep), *sleep-maintenance insomnia* (waking up frequently during the night and being unable to get back to sleep within fifteen minutes), and *early-morning awakening insomnia* (waking up too early and not being able to fall back asleep). And, as if all that wasn't complicated enough, there's also *mixed insomnia*, which is a combination of these problems.

How do I deal with insomnia?

First, realize that you're not alone. About 74 percent of the adult population experience insomnia at least a few nights per week. The good news is there are cures for your problem.

Research suggests that the best way to control chronic insomnia is with a combination of prescription sleep medications (such as benzodiazepines, non-benzodiazepines, and ramelteon) along with behavioral treatments. The medications provide immediate relief while cognitive behavior therapy (CBT) ideally supplies the long-term solution. CBT has five main components:

Stimulus control. This involves removing anything from the bedroom that might disrupt sleep, such as computers, television sets, video games, telephones, Blackberrys, work-related material, dirty clothes, photos of your mother-in-law … The goal is to make your bedroom into a distraction- and angst-free sanctuary that is designed for one thing: peaceful sleep.

Sleep restriction. Many insomniacs spend so much time tossing and turning that they come to associate their bed with sleeplessness. This behavioral technique is designed to break that psychological association by having patients stay up until they're so tired that they fall asleep immediately when their head hits the pillow. This is done for a few nights, and then bedtime is gradually moved up.

Relaxation training. You can learn to control and quiet your nervous system, thus helping your mind get into a better mood for sleep. This is done through simple breathing and muscle-relaxation exercises that reduce overall body tension. Imagining tranquil scenes and pleasant moments is also a part of it.

Cognitive psychotherapy. A big part of beating insomnia is becoming less anxious about it. Instead of dreading going to sleep and worrying about how you're going to function the next day, psychotherapy helps replace negative thoughts with positive ones and enables you to be less concerned about nights when sleep is more difficult.

Sleep hygiene education. This involves examining and, if necessary, changing eating habits, caffeine and alcohol consumption, exercise routines, and even styles of bedroom drapes or sheets. Sometimes a simple adjustment such as having five minutes of "worry time" just before bed, or turning the alarm clock away from you so the digital numbers don't taunt you all night, will make a big difference.

According to Carlos Schenck, MD, of the Minnesota Regional Sleep Disorders Center and one of the most renowned experts in the field: "Whatever you do, don't let insomnia become an accepted way of life. Seek medical attention if the problem becomes frequent; there may be an underlying medical or psychological condition causing your sleep problem, or you may just need some help getting back to a healthful sleep routine. There are many remedies available to remind you of what it feels like to get a good night's sleep."

SLEEP APNEA

My spouse says I snore loudly and occasionally even stop breathing. I'm unaware of any of this but am exhausted during the day. Should I be worried?

It sounds as though you have obstructive sleep apnea (OSA), another common disorder. Get to your doctor immediately because, if left untreated for any length of time, it can be life threatening. OSA is characterized by pauses in breathing during sleep. Your respiratory passages collapse and become constricted, stopping airflow to your lungs. These pauses can last up to ten seconds and may occur seven hundred times throughout the night. Because you're waking up each time to resume breathing, you can see why you're so tired the next day. People with OSA are often oblivious of these interruptions, which include heavy snoring, having no idea why they wake up with severe dry mouth and suffer daytime drowsiness, impaired memory and concentration, and even high blood pressure and depression.

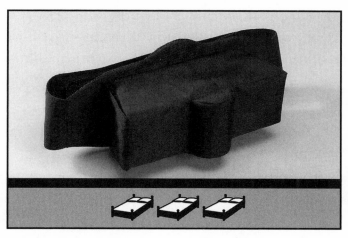

Zzoma, a belt-like device worn during sleep, alleviates positional sleep apnea, including some snoring.

Are some people more at risk of sleep apnea than others?

Eighteen percent of the adult population has sleep apnea, and 95 percent of them don't know it. Two times as many men have OSA than women. Obesity increases the risk and is a predominant trait in most sufferers. In fact, the more overweight you are, the more likely it is you'll have it. Any male whose neck size is greater than 17 ½ inches is a likely candidate. Other risk factors include old age, menopause, smoking, asthma, enlarged tonsils, and a previously broken nose.

What should I do if I think I have sleep apnea?

Ask your family physician for a referral to an accredited sleep disorders center. This usually involves spending a night in the sleep lab being monitored for respiration and heart-rate issues. In the meantime, try:

- Losing weight if you're carrying a few extra pounds.

- Avoiding alcohol and sedatives. (These suppress the body's mechanism that wakes you up when you stop breathing.)

- Changing your sleeping position. Because OSA is often worse when lying on your back, try putting a tennis ball in a sock and pinning it to the back of your nightshirt. This will help keep you on your side, although it may drive your cocker spaniel crazy.

Are there any non-surgical treatment options?

The most recommended and effective non-surgical treatment for sleep apnea is a Continuous Positive Airway Pressure (CPAP) machine. To use it, you must wear a plastic mask over your nose (and sometimes mouth) while sleeping in order to receive a flow of pressurized air to the back of the throat. This keeps your airway passages open by facilitating inhaling. The drawback? Well, besides making it challenging to be romantic, the CPAP can be uncomfortable. However, when

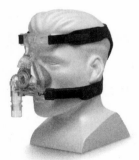

ComfortGel Nasal Mask

Used with permission of Respironics, Inc., Murrysville, PA

CPAP devices can make breathing at night easier.

used properly, it has a 70 percent success rate—dramatically reducing the risk of heart attack, minimizing daytime drowsiness, lessening the chance of falling asleep while driving, counteracting depression, and generally improving quality of life. So you don't look like George Clooney in pajamas? Big deal.

A less-intrusive alternative for those with mild OSA is a fitted, plastic device that slips over the teeth. By keeping your jaw and tongue forward and elevating your soft palate while you're sleeping, it opens the upper airway and minimizes symptoms. Patients who go this route should have regular dental checkups.

What about surgery?

While it's tempting to look for a remedy that isn't as cumbersome as the CPAP and oral devices, be careful. There are many risks involved, and the procedures often have low success rates. Here's what's out there, but before pursuing any one, get a second opinion:

- *Uvulopaltopharyngoplasty (UPPP)* is the most common surgery. Excess tissue is removed from the back of the throat and the soft palate in order to widen the airway. The tonsils are also removed. This operation reduces snoring and helps 40 percent to 45 percent of patients—although most will never be able to pronounce it.

- *Temperature-controlled, radio-frequency, tongue-based reduction* involves using needle electrodes to shrink and stiffen upper airway tissue, thus promoting better airflow. It is somewhat effective.

- *Jaw and facial surgery* is another treatment option, in which the upper and lower jaws are cut and repositioned more forward, providing additional room for the tongue and reducing the likelihood of it blocking the airway. The success rate can be 90 percent but depends a great deal on the experience of the surgeon.

- *Tracheostomy* is done only in extreme cases. A breathing tube is inserted into the trachea through an opening in the front of the neck, thereby bypassing the upper airway obstruction. At night the valve is opened. This treatment is 100 percent effective, but for obvious reasons it can interfere with quality of life.

RESTLESS LEGS SYNDROME

Sometimes I get unpleasant sensations in my legs at night, and the only way I can get relief is by moving around. What's going on?

You probably have Restless Legs Syndrome (RLS). It's the third most common sleep disorder, affecting 10 percent to 15 percent of the population and about 30 percent to 40 percent of older adults. Approximately 26 percent of pregnant women get RLS, and it often worsens in the months preceding childbirth. Sufferers usually experience sensations of warmth, pain, pulling, deep itching, or even feeling as though insects are crawling beneath the skin. About 70 percent of patients suffer from leg twitches every twenty to forty seconds throughout the night. Often the only way to make these sensations go away is to move the legs or get up and walk around. The more you try to ignore the symptoms the worse they tend to get. RLS may be primary, meaning there's no underlying disorder causing it, or secondary, meaning another condition or medication is to blame. In most cases it's a lifelong affliction, but it can be managed.

What can I do to treat RLS?

The first step is getting a simple blood test to determine if deficiencies in vitamin B12, iron, or folic acid are causing it. If that's the case, then increasing your consumption of those things may remedy it. Otherwise, medications such as Requip® and Merapex®, in addition to lifestyle changes such as avoiding caffeine and alcohol and exercising moderately at night, can have positive effects. Because it is generally a long-term affliction, sufferers should approach it as such with ongoing checkups and doctor oversight.

NARCOLEPSY

Talk about weird. Sometimes I'll get weak and actually collapse after laughing or being frightened. I'm also excessively tired during the day. What's happening?

You've just described two of the four most common symptoms of a disorder called narcolepsy. Excessive daytime drowsiness occurs even after a good night's rest and causes the sufferer to nod off throughout

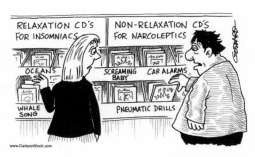

the day. The loss of muscle control is known as "cataplexy" and is usually triggered by a strong emotion or shock. The person remains aware during the episode, which usually lasts no more than five minutes. Approximately 70 percent of narcoleptics experience cataplexy.

What's happening is that your body's boundaries between sleep and wakefulness have become blurred, and this has serious physical, psychological, and social ramifications. Narcolepsy is highly associated with dysfunctions in REM sleep, and about 0.05 percent of the American population suffers from it. It typically begins during puberty but often takes ten to fifteen years to be properly diagnosed. The disorder runs in families.

Okay, I'm batting .500. What are the other two symptoms?

- *Hypnagogic (and hypnopompic) hallucinations* often arise because sufferers tend to enter REM within minutes of falling asleep and start dreaming immediately. This makes it difficult for narcoleptics to differentiate between "sleep-onset" dreams and reality. The experiences can be vague, scary, odd, and disorienting. Hypnagogic hallucinations occur while falling asleep, while hypnopompic hallucinations occur when awakening.

- *Sleep paralysis* occurs when the brain is awake but the body is not. Therefore, you feel as though you're unable to move. The feeling can arrive when you're falling asleep or waking up, and it may be accompanied by hallucinations and a sense of doom or panic. Actually, many people who are sleep-deprived but not narcoleptic experience this phenomenon.

Only 10 percent to 25 percent of those with narcolepsy suffer from all four symptoms.

How can narcolepsy be treated?

This is a job for your doctor or a sleep professional. Although there is no cure, a combination of medications can help you manage it. Treatment usually begins with Modafinil because it helps people stay awake and is relatively safe and user-friendly. Stimulants are occasionally prescribed to boost alertness, but their use needs to be carefully monitored due to potentially negative side effects. Antidepressants, such as selective serotonin reuptake inhibitors and tricyclic antidepressants, are also sometimes prescribed to control cataplexy.

CIRCADIAN RHYTHM DISORDERS

Why don't I ever feel tired until 2:00 or 3:00 AM?

You might be suffering from something called delayed sleep phase disorder (DSPD). It's caused by your body clock or circadian rhythm being out of synch with the rest of the world. This happens to everyone periodically because of shift work, jetlag, or just partying late on the weekends, but it's considered chronic when your normal sleep/wake schedule is routinely at least two hours later than conventional and interferes with job, family, and social responsibilities. On average, the disorder starts at age twenty and occurs among 7 percent to 16 percent of the population. Most often it involves difficulty getting to sleep at a "normal" hour and then having trouble getting up in the morning in time for work and appointments. Over time, you can build up a sizable sleep debt and experience daytime drowsiness. Approximately 40 percent of those with DSPD have a family history of the problem.

Conversely, advanced sleep phase disorder (ASPD) occurs when you have a strong propensity to go to sleep (and subsequently awaken) earlier than conventional. Even though you may be getting eight hours or more of quality sleep, if it significantly disrupts your life then you may need treatment.

Can anything be done about DSPD (or ASPD)?

The most effective treatment for both of these disorders is light therapy. Those with DSPD should expose themselves to either natural or artificial daylight spectrum light earlier in the day and dim the lights at least two hours before a normal bedtime in order to advance their body clocks. Less light exposure in the evening promotes the production of melatonin, our natural sleepy-time hormone. Those with ASPD should do the opposite, keeping the drapes drawn later in the morning and the lights on later at night.

Another treatment for Circadian Rhythm Disorders is chronotherapy. A DSPD sufferer, for example, would stay up two to three hours later on successive nights (while keeping their total amount of sleep time constant) until they eventually work their way around the clock and reach the desired bedtime. This is fairly impractical, though, unless you want to spend your vacation getting your sleep schedule in order.

SLEEPWALKING

Does this really happen?

Without a doubt. Sleepwalking is a state of partial arousal where the brain is awake while other parts of the body are asleep. People who sleepwalk are able to carry out complex actions without any awareness of what they're doing. Sleepwalking is unpredictable, and episodes can range from just walking round the bedroom to strolling out of the house or even driving a car. Sleepwalkers will normally have a blank expression 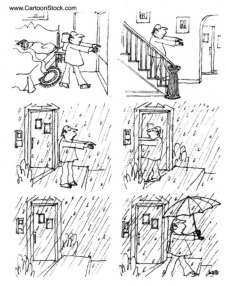 or a glassy-eyed stare, and be disoriented if awakened. Only about 4 percent of adults are sleepwalkers. In the majority of cases (65 percent), genetic factors are responsible. For the rest, sleep deprivation is usually the cause.

Children are actually the biggest group of sleepwalkers. Around 17 percent will have episodes, most commonly at ages eleven and twelve. It's considered a normal part of development, however, and usually doesn't require medical intervention.

How is sleepwalking treated?

- Make sure you regularly get the appropriate amount of sleep each night.

- If your child regularly sleepwalks, wake him shortly before the time when it usually happens for several consecutive nights to break the pattern. Don't worry, you won't have to stay up until dawn; sleepwalking tends to occur in the first third of the night.

- Self-hypnosis has been successful with mild cases. It involves reaching a state of altered consciousness where you're very receptive to orders because attention is highly focused and critical thinking has been reduced. The "orders" are initially given by the therapist, with instructions to the patient on how to trigger the same thoughts independently.

- A class of prescription drugs called Benzodiazepines are often prescribed for particularly worrisome and potentially dangerous cases. They're very effective in controlling sleepwalking and generally safe for long-term use, as is clonazepam.

If there's a sleepwalker in the house, what safety measures should I take?

A door alarm may be a good idea in order to wake up the sleepwalker or to alert the rest of the household. You should try to confine him to the ground floor and make sure all windows are locked. Weapons should not be easily accessible anywhere in the house and especially in the bedroom. If you find someone sleepwalking, the best thing to do is quietly direct him back to bed without waking him up.

SLEEP TALKING

Do I have a problem if I talk in my sleep?

Only if you're divulging state secrets to beautiful Russian spies. And even in that case, you could argue that science has shown that sleep talking is not a product of a conscious or rational mind. It can occur during any stage of sleep and

> You may be communicating in more ways than just speech while you sleep. It has been shown that it is possible to send e-mail while sleeping. Gmail's Mail Goggles feature tests your ability to solve math problems before letting you send e-mail late at night.

can range from incoherent mumbling to involved dialogue. Sleep talkers are unaware of their behavior, and their voice/language may differ from what they normally use. Once again, children are the biggest group of sufferers (it affects 50 percent), but there are no negative consequences other than disrupting the sleep of others in the room or house.

SLEEP EATING

When and why does this happen?

Someone with sleep-related eating disorder (SRED) may get out of bed and raid the fridge or attempt to ingest food, drink, or even something inedible that's close at hand. Some may even prepare complex meals (although they usually stop short of doing the dishes). It all stems from a strong urge to eat, regardless of whether they're hungry. Individual levels of consciousness and memory vary greatly. It affects about 1 percent of the American population, with three out of four sufferers being women.

How is it treated?

The medication topiramate is usually prescribed for SRED. Other types of treatments include hypnotherapy, biofeedback, acupuncture, psychotherapy, and behavioral strategies. Quitting smoking, controlling substance abuse, and reducing stress can also work.

SLEEP TERRORS (NIGHT TERRORS)

Why does my son sit up in bed and scream?

He's probably experiencing what's called a "night terror." These usually occur during the first half of sleep and are generally characterized by a racing heart, fast breathing, increased sweating, heightened blood pressure, and dilated pupils. People with sleep terrors normally have an intense desire to escape or an impulse to fight the perceived attack with great strength and speed. Sleep terrors and sleepwalking frequently afflict the same person. Episodes are typically only a few minutes long, and the person often resumes normal sleeping with no memory of the event.

Who is most likely to suffer from sleep terrors?

Boys between the ages of three and twelve. (Only 2 percent of adults suffer them.) Sleep terrors seem to run in families, but they can be precipitated by stress, sleep deprivation, and a full bladder. Additionally, in females, menstrual periods and alcohol use can bring them on in adulthood. Scary movies usually don't help either.

What should I do?

Comfort him as best you can. Sleep terrors generally pose no threat and disappear with time. If they are particularly severe, benzodiazepine medications are often effective, along with occasional low doses of antidepressants. Alternative treatments include psychotherapy and stress reduction. Self-hypnosis and visual imagery techniques are also good for treating children and adults with sleep terrors and sleepwalking.

SLEEP PARALYSIS

Sometimes I wake up, and I'm unable to move. What's going on?

This is a disorder called sleep paralysis. You're unable to move from head to toe, apart from the eyes, and there may also be labored breathing, a feeling of fear, and a sense that something or someone is in the room. Some people also experience tingling or shaking sensations, bursts of light, tunnel vision, buzzing sounds, or feel like they're floating. This can last anywhere from thirty seconds to five minutes.

Sleep paralysis may arise as a symptom of narcolepsy, but it can also appear on its own, in which case it's called recurrent isolated sleep paralysis. Approximately 25 percent to 30 percent of the population will experience this at least once during their lifetime.

What factors make someone susceptible to sleep paralysis?

Anyone who is sleep-deprived, feverish, or aroused from a deep sleep may experience it. Adolescents are particularly at risk, as are shift workers and the overly anxious. But even simple things like your sleep position can trigger it. Those who sleep on their backs are five times more at risk.

What should I do if it happens to me?

Don't panic. It is not a sign of some underlying neurological condition and, in most cases, it will probably never happen again. If it does become chronic, however, or if you develop a fear of it reoccurring that prevents you from getting a good night's rest, then:

- Avoid daytime naps.
- Sleep on your side.
- Make small movements instead of large ones when trying to break the paralysis.
- Cough
- Go back to sleep.
- Relax by telling yourself you know what's happening and that it's benign.

REM SLEEP BEHAVIOR DISORDER

I've recently started having vivid confrontational dreams that, according to my wife, I violently act out. What does this mean?

You're experiencing REM Sleep Behavior Disorder (RBD). Although it affects just 0.5 percent of the population, 85 percent are men over age fifty. RBD produces vivid, intense, physically active, confrontational, aggressive, and violent dreams that often contain fight-or-flight scenarios. Although this may sound more entertaining than an episode of *Cops*, it can be dangerous to yourself and your bed partner depending on how active you get. Ninety percent of those with RBD remember the dreams and, despite the energy expended, aren't overly tired during the day.

What should I do to control them?

Chronic RBD rarely gets better by itself, so see a sleep specialist as soon as possible. In 90 percent of cases, the drug clonazepam is effective. Melatonin- and dopamine-enhancing medications may also help. There is some evidence that RBD could be a precursor to neurodegenerative diseases like Alzheimer's and Parkinson's disease.

SEXOMNIA

My husband occasionally wakes me up by aggressively trying to have sex with me, but I think he's asleep. How can this be?

This is what's known as sleepsex, or sexomnia. It's a disorder that can include making sexual sounds, masturbating, fondling, and intercourse. And, yes, the person is asleep and completely unaware of what he/she is doing. In fact, partners are often embarrassed, disturbed, or even disbelieving when told about it in the morning. It can occur with both men and women, is caused by OSA (obstructive sleep apnea) and can be controlled using a CPAP device.

When it happens within a committed relationship, such behavior can be aggravating, exasperating, and, depending on how aggressive it is, even threatening. But it can really become a problem—with potential criminal consequences—when a sufferer is sharing a hotel room or spending the night at a friend's home and has an episode. Molestation, rape, unwanted pregnancy, and the transmission of sexual disease are all possible.

How to Treat Sexomnia

Sexomnia appears to be controlled by an obscure, internal, hair-trigger alarm mechanism that sends a person out of NREM (non-rapid eye movement) sleep and into a confused quasi-awake state. This is called disordered arousal. But what causes this alarm to sound is unknown. Sleepsex seems to arise without any particular cause. However, there are a few precautions that can be taken to reduce its likelihood:

- Reduce alcohol intake to a minimum.

- Ensure that you get a sufficient amount of sleep each night.

- Don't sleep in the nude and wear pajamas that are difficult to remove.

- Lock bedroom doors.

- Don't share a bed with a child or an unsuspecting friend.

- If you tend to talk loudly during sexomnia, sleep with the radio on in order to cut down on gossip in your apartment complex.

- Clonazepam is 90 percent effective in controlling sexomnia.

OTHER RESOURCES

There are several books that focus in depth on sleep disorders. One of the best is *Sleep: A Groundbreaking Guide to the Mysteries, the Problems, and the Solutions* by Carlos H. Schenck.

When to Seek Help

If you're routinely robbed of a good night's rest, you may have a sleep disorder. This chart lists symptoms associated with several common sleep problems. For each symptom you have, decide how severely or how frequently it affects you, on a 10-point scale. Then check the chart to see whether you should seek treatment. If you experience two or more symptoms, consider moving up to the next recommendation level.

If your family doctor's suggested remedies don't improve your sleep after a reasonable period, or if your main problem is daytime sleepiness, ask for a referral to a sleep-disorders center for an evaluation.

Symptoms	very mild 1	2	3	4	5	6	7	8	9	10 severe
Gasp, choke, or stop breathing during sleep										
Snore loudly; have high blood pressure; overweight										
Feel creeping, crawling sensations in legs while lying down										
Feel tired and sleepy while driving										
Arms and legs jerk and twitch during sleep										
Wake up at night; feel fatigued during the day										
Fall asleep in front of the TV or while reading during day or early evening										
Wake up tired and lethargic in the morning										
Experience disturbing nightmares										
Have occasional sleeplessness at home and during trips										

Treatment needed? Not necessarily   Recommended   Definitely

Source: Dr. Michael J. Thorpy, director, Sleep-Wake Disorders Center, Montefiore Medical Center, New York City.

Figure 13.1. When to seek help. Copyright 1997 by Consumers Union of U.S., Inc. Yonkers, NY 10703-1057, a nonprofit organization. Reprinted with permission from the March 1996 issue of Consumer Reports® for educational purposes only. No commercial use or reproduction permitted. www.ConsumerReports.org.

Fig. 4 When to seek help. Courtesy Dr. Michael J. Thorpy, Sleep Wake Disorders Center, Montefiore Medical Center, New York City

18

Knock Yourself Out: Sleep Drugs

We take pills to make us healthy, boost our mood, keep us focused, and even to have better sex. If it comes in tablet form and promises to help us feel even a little better, most people will swallow it. And it's no different with sleep. About one in every two Americans experience occasional insomnia, and nearly one in four suffer from it every or almost every night. Although only 10 percent of adults report taking sleep aids, between 2001 and 2005 prescriptions for sleeping pills increased by 60 percent and are still on the rise. There are hundreds of prescriptions, over-the-counter, and herbal options available today that promise to knock you out and keep you out. This chapter is designed to help you understand and sort through them all, whether you're looking for something to pop before a long flight in coach or to take the anxious edge off a difficult day. In some ways, this is the chapter of last resort—the place you turn when more holistic suggestions don't work. But it's also the area where you must tread most cautiously, because some of these pills have serious side effects and can actually make matters worse.

Drug tolerance: Over time, you may have to increase the dosage of the medication to continue to feel any effect. This could have you popping pills and paying bills more frequently than you'd like.

Drug dependence: You may eventually become dependent on whatever you're taking—psychologically or physiologically. This can actually worsen your sleep.

Withdrawal symptoms: If you suddenly stop taking some drugs, you may experience nausea, trembling, sweating, or additional sleeping problems.

Drug interactions: Mixing other medications or alcohol with sleep aids can worsen symptoms and side effects and even cause death.

Masking root problems: Poor sleep may be the result of an undiagnosed health problem. So by taking a sleeping pill, you're really just treating a symptom.

Side effects: These drugs have many, which we'll discuss.

STOP! If You Fit Into One of These Categories, Don't Take Sleep Meds.

People with Emergency Jobs (such as on-call doctors or volunteer firefighters)

Why not? Some drugs cause mental impairment or drowsiness when a person suddenly wakes. Most sleep aids are recommended only to be taken when you have a solid, guaranteed seven to nine hours of sleep time ahead of you.

What else can I try? Consult your doctor about which drugs require that continuous sleep window and ensure that no drug you take will make you impaired or drowsy if you suddenly have to get up. If at all possible, turn to behavioral therapy as your first solution.

Pregnant or Nursing Moms

Why not? A mother should consider anything she puts into her body as something she's sharing with her child. Drugs that Mom takes can enter the placenta or breast milk and affect the baby; some can even cause birth defects. Most drugs have never been tested on pregnant mothers.

What else can I try? For pregnant moms, comfort is key! Check out our recommendations for a comfortable bedroom environment, stress relief, and solutions to insomnia. When nursing, try to match your sleep schedule with your baby's so you are getting consistent, regular sleep. Nap when baby naps and only do chores when baby is awake.

Those with Sleep Apnea

Why not? Sleep apnea is a breathing problem; it literally means "sleep without breath." Some drugs make breathing even more difficult, thereby putting a person with sleep apnea at higher risk of dangerous, belabored breathing at night.

What else can I try? Consult your doctor and do your research on any drugs you're considering. Make sure it doesn't involve any side effects or chemicals that could affect your ability to breathe or the diameter of your air passageways. But, as always, we recommend first trying behavioral therapy and of course investing in a CPAP machine. (CPAP stands for **C**ontinuous **P**ositive **A**irway **P**ressure; it's the most commonly prescribed treatment for sleep apnea).

History of Drug or Alcohol Abuse

Why not? Sleep drugs are, in fact, drugs. Some are addictive, and a history of drug or alcohol addiction can increase your risk of becoming dependent on the pill.

What else can I try? We always recommend behavioral therapy as the first solution. Return to the chapters that discuss your specific sleep problem and be persistent in giving our tricks a shot. If you *must* turn to sleep aids, be extra cautious about the risks of addiction for each medication.

Under 18 Years

Why not? There isn't a single sleep drug that's been FDA approved for child use. In fact, benzodiazepines are specifically recommended to *not* be used on children.

What else can I try? Behavioral techniques such as regular sleep schedules and bedtime routines seem to work well with children. Enforce rules like no caffeine, no electronics, and no stimulating activities before bedtime. For more tips, review Chapter 9.

Sleeping pills are just as serious a drug as any other, and they need to be treated as such!

Here are some general guidelines for using sleep aids:

1. Call the doctor. As with any drug, you first need to understand what you're taking and whether it's right for you. This usually means talking to your physician or, better yet, a doctor who specializes in sleep medicine. Make sure he or she is aware of all medications, vitamins, and supplements you're taking, as well as past health problems.

2. Follow the rules. While talking to a professional is a vital first step, you have to follow through by taking any prescribed medication as directed. Most sleeping pills must be swallowed on an empty stomach a specific amount of time before you hope to fall asleep. Each brand is different, though, so you have to follow instructions.

3. Check the clock. One of the most important things to keep in mind is that you should only take these drugs when you have seven to nine hours to rest. If you need to drive somewhere, give an important presentation, take an exam, or do some complex task sooner than that, don't make the mistake of thinking you'll be able to pop one of these and be at your best. You may be groggy or dizzy when you wake up.

What are my options?

Five Popular Herbal Remedies: Herbal remedies are intriguing options because they're more natural than their pill-form counterparts. But keep in mind that herbal remedies are *not* regulated by the FDA, so it's buyer beware!

Name	Also Called	What It Is	Potential Side Effects	How It's Used
Melatonin	n/a	A hormone secreted by the pineal gland in the brain; helps induce sleep and increase its duration; levels are higher at night than during the day	Headaches, confusion, drowsiness, fatigue, vivid dreams, hypothermia, upset stomach, and retinal damage	Taken as a dietary supplement in tablet form, doses range from 0.1-10mg, most typically 3-5mg
Valerian Root	Valerian Officinalis	A plant that supposedly shortens the amount of time it takes to fall asleep and reduces nighttime awakenings	Headaches, excitability, heart disturbances, ataxia, hypothermia, muscle relaxation, and morning grogginess	Can be taken as an oral capsule or as a crude root; crude root dosages typically range between 2-10g per day
5-HTP	5-Hydroxytryptophan Ditropan Apo-Oxybutynin Oxbutyn	A derivative of the amino acid tryptophan; immediate precursor to the hormone serotonin which helps induce sleep	Some studies have shown no benefit of taking 5-HTP; side effects include nausea, dry mouth, constipation, esophagitis, urinary hesitancy, flushing, and urticaria	Found in certain foods like cheese and white-meat poultry; can also be taken in supplement forms of 50-100mg gelatin or vegetarian capsules
Chamomile	Literally means "earth-apple"	A daisy-like plant that is said to have anti-inflammatory and anti-bacterial properties; also shown to relieve anxiety and stress	Possible allergic reaction, vomiting; in pregnant women, could lead to stimulation of the uterus and abortion	Available as capsules, liquid, extracts, teas, and topical creams, among other preparations
Kava Kava	Awa Kew Tonga	An ancient plant (dried rhizome and roots) used for non-addictive stress and anxiety relief; also said to relax muscles and induce sleep	Mild euphoria, happiness, fluent/lively speech, possibly hepatitis, cirrhosis, and liver failure; increases toxicity of alcohol	Steep pulverized root in hot water, filter, and drink

If melatonin is a natural hormone, why is it so controversial?

Melatonin is regarded as a food supplement in the United States and, therefore, not regulated by the FDA. This means that there are no assurances that what you're buying is pure or will work as promised. In fact, both Canada and the UK banned melatonin because not enough is known about it. Furthermore, there's limited study of its effects on children, and it can be dangerous to people with Type I diabetes because it impacts glucose tolerance.

> Melatonin was first discovered by its ability to change the skin color of amphibians and reptiles.

On a more positive note, a number of scientists have suggested that melatonin might help slow the aging process. Various research has shown some correlation with age and the decrease of melatonin. Perhaps this is why the elderly generally have more problems sleeping. Because melatonin is produced most readily in the dark, regulating your light exposure may be a good natural way to boost your own melatonin or prevent its decrease as you age.

Are there any totally safe and effective natural drugs?

Yes. L-tryptophan, or simply tryptophan, is a close relative of melatonin that is found in many foods and can help induce sleep. Here's a quick chemistry lesson (we apologize) to help you understand how it works:

L-Tryptophan—(is converted to)→ 5-HTP—(is converted to)→ Serotonin—(is converted to)→ Melatonin—(helps induce)→ Sleep!

Ever wonder why you're so tired after a Thanksgiving meal? It's probably due to the fact that turkey contains lots of L-tryptophan. Other sources of L-tryptophan include chocolate, eggs, fish, bananas, milk, poultry, yogurt, and more.

Four Popular Over-the-Counter Drugs

When people hear OTC sleep drugs, they usually think of antihistamines and allergy medicines. That's because these drugs all produce a sedative effect. Their active ingredients are typically Doxylamine or Diphenhydramine. OTC drugs are popular choices because they're cheap and accessible, but unless you want to head to the drugstore each week for the rest of your life buying allergy medicine to fall asleep, these are only a *temporary* solution. Use them only when you're going through a "rough patch" of sleep (that long international flight or anxiety-ridden night), and in all other cases rely on behavioral therapy.

Benadryl is an antihistamine used to treat sneezing, runny nose, and allergies. It's also commonly used to induce sleep. You should use caution when taking it—it's known to cause dizziness and confusion and may be dangerous while driving or doing anything physical. It can also cause headaches and dry mouth. Take this approximately thirty minutes before bed.

Nytol is an antihistamine used to treat occasional sleeplessness. Like similar medicines, it may cause dizziness. But in addition, it may also make you more susceptible to sunburns and can cause fainting if combined with exercise and hot weather. Not all stores carry this brand, but a generic one can be substituted.

Sominex allows from six to eight hours of sleep but warns of potential dizziness and drowsiness. It claims *not* to be habit-forming if used for short spans of time, and also claims to be the "doctor-preferred" sleep aid.

Tylenol PM is used for temporary relief from aches and pains with accompanying sleeplessness. It's available in many forms: rapid-release gels, vanilla liquid, caplets, and geltabs. It warns of drowsiness and recommends that you don't drink alcohol or operate a motor vehicle while on the drug.

Four Popular Prescription Drugs

The *non-benzodiazepines*, otherwise known as "Z-drugs," have become very popular in the prescription arena. Although expensive, these sleeping pills help you fall asleep and stay asleep, and they include some of the newest drugs on the market. Benzodiazepines, on the other hand, such as the prescription drugs Ativan and Valium, act as a depressant on the central nervous system to lull you to sleep. Here are the pros and cons of the top four in this category:

Ambien

The Pros: Claims to "help you fall asleep fast and stay asleep" • FDA-approved • Non-narcotic • Recommended for both common and chronic insomnia • Covered by most insurance companies.

The Cons: Side effects include headaches, dizziness, and "amnesia," where the user may not remember what happens several hours after taking the pill • Beware of tolerance problems, dependence, withdrawal symptoms, and unusual changes in behavior such as confusion, aggression, agitation, hallucinations, and suicidal thoughts • Particularly risky for pregnant women.

> **Ambien Amnesia**
>
> In an article headlined, "Some Sleeping Pill Users Range Far Beyond Bed," *New York Times* reporter Stephanie Saul tells the story of a registered nurse who took Ambien before going to bed one night. After falling asleep, she went out into the 20-degree Denver night wearing only a thin nightshirt, got into her car, caused an accident, urinated in the intersection, and then got into a violent altercation with police who tried to arrest her. She claims to remember nothing about what happened.

Rozerem

The Pros: Claims little-to-no risk of drug dependence or abuse • FDA-approved • Targets receptors in the brain that control your twenty-four-hour clock • Sedative used to treat common insomnia.

The Cons: Side effects include dizziness, headache, stuffy nose, nausea, diarrhea, and sore throat • Particularly risky for those with liver disease.

Sonata

The Pros: Claims to be a hypnotic agent giving relief for millions from sleeplessness • FDA-approved for short-term use • Beneficial for people who haven't taken a sleeping pill at bedtime but who wake up during the middle of the night and want to sleep one to three more hours. (Most sleeping pills make users sleepy for at least eight hours.)

The Cons: Not very beneficial for people who struggle to *stay* asleep (as opposed to *fall* asleep) • Side effects include drowsiness, amnesia, withdrawal, and difficulty with coordination.

Lunesta

The Pros: Claims "while some sleep aids help you fall asleep and some help you stay asleep, Lunesta has been proven to do both, so you can get a full night of sleep" • Claims lower risk of tolerance buildup and insomnia rebound (which means a worsening of insomnia when taken off the drug) • FDA-approved • Non-narcotic.

The Cons: Side effects include a bad taste in your mouth, drowsiness, dizziness, headache, and cold symptoms • More serious side effects include memory loss, anxiety, allergic reactions, and abnormal thoughts (such as aggressive, confused, agitated, depressed, and even suicidal thoughts).

> **It's in the headlines!**
>
> According to *Men's Health* magazine, "Unlike its chemical cousins Sonata and Ambien, which tend to lose their potency toward morning, Lunesta is effective throughout the sleep cycle—without disrupting the critical deep stages. It put our guinea pig to sleep in record time, kept him there for eight hours, and left him feeling wide-eyed and alert the next day."

Note: All prescription drugs are required to list ingredients. If you find an ingredient ending in "amine," it could mean damaging effects on sleep quality.

> ### Insomniac Michael Jackson Begged for Sedative
>
> Michael Jackson took more than ten Xanax pills a night, asking his employees to get the prescription medicine under their names and also personally traveling to doctors' offices in other states to obtain them. The insomniac singer traveled with an anesthesiologist who would "take him down" at night and "bring him back up" during a world tour in the mid nineties.

How common are side-effects of sleep aids?

It's very common to have mild side effects from sleeping pills, most commonly dizziness, drowsiness, headaches, dry mouth or throat, and diarrhea. Keep in mind that side effects vary from person to person, though, and that many people are able to control them and get a great night of sleep. The key is *making sure* the medication is right for you and *following directions* when you take it.

What should I take if I have …?

Insomnia: difficulty in falling or staying asleep; can be transient or chronic.

Solution: because insomnias vary greatly between people, you may be able to use any of the solutions discussed thus far in this chapter depending on what your doctor recommends and what's right for you.

Parasomnias: arousals from Stage 4 sleep including sleepwalking, sleeptalking, night terrors, teeth grinding, Restless Legs Syndrome, and periodic limb movement disorder.

Solution: Only consider medication when the episodes are long-lasting and frequent. Benzodiazepines, a specific group of drugs that depress the central nervous system, are commonly recommended for such sleep disorders. Mirapex specifically works well for Restless Legs Syndrome. Other commonly used benzodiazepines are Klonopin,

Valium, and Restoril. Benzodiazepines are generally safe in the short term but are not recommended for long-term use or use by pregnant women and children under eighteen.

Sleep Rhythm Disorders: any irregular sleep and wake schedule, including delayed sleep phase, advanced sleep phase, shift-work sleep disorder, and jetlag.

Solution: Melatonin can sometimes be helpful in regulating your sleep schedule because it affects your circadian rhythm, or the "human clock" that keeps you running in twenty-four-hour cycles. Be aware of its risks, however, which we discussed earlier. Before turning to this supplement, try regulating your light exposure naturally to induce the production of melatonin in your brain.

What does the future hold?

Since so many people are having difficulty sleeping, there's lots of money and effort being spent on finding that magic pill. Currently, there are about a half dozen drugs in the works. One area of particular interest and promise involves a neurotransmitter called GABA. It appears to encourage sedation by slowing the fight-or-flight response prevalent in so many of us twenty-first-century adrenaline junkies.

Sleeping aids may not be right for you and, in general, it's best to think of them as a last resort. There is substantial evidence that the combination of sleeping pills and cognitive behavioral therapy (CBT), or CBT alone, is more effective in the long run than just taking pills. But if you experiment and find the perfect pill, it can mean the difference between a sleepy existence and a more alert, happy life.

19 Personal Observations

Jim Maas

Having finished researching and writing *Sleep for Success!*, I've been reminiscing about my last forty years studying sleep. I was hooked for good on a November night (not particularly dark and stormy) way back in 1969. I was visiting Dr. William C. Dement at Stanford University. Bill is now recognized as the undisputed father of modern-day sleep research.

At that time I was an assistant professor at Cornell University and making films to enhance my lectures for teaching introductory psychology. There weren't any audio/visual materials that focused on sleep, even though that activity (or lack thereof) occupies almost one-third of our lives. And the topic of sleep was only briefly mentioned in psych textbooks—maybe just a few paragraphs. Indeed, the science of sleep was in its infancy.

Bill Dement and his former colleagues at the University of Chicago, Nathaniel Kleitman and Eugene Aserinsky, had only recently discovered that rapid eye movements (REMs) occurred at various times during sleep. These signaled that the sleeper was probably dreaming. This remarkable finding turned out to be the key that unlocked the theater of the night. It would ultimately lead to a proliferation of sleep research, the field of sleep medicine, and the establishment of centers for the treatment of sleep disorders—but I'm getting ahead of my story.

I wanted to witness firsthand (and film) how Bill Dement "captured" dreams in the sleep laboratory. Observing his all-night sleep-recording session was so captivating that it altered the course of my career. Watching an instrument make a mile-long paper recording of the brain wave and eye movement activity of a "wired-up" sleeping graduate assistant named Steve might not sound exactly riveting, but to me it was life changing.

Before Steve fell asleep, his brain waves were fast; the polygraph's pens moved vigorously. Thirty minutes after sleep onset, the waves were slower and eye movements had all but ceased, indicating deep sleep. I was in the control room struggling to remain awake, suffering from jetlag and being hypnotized by the rhythmic slow scratches of the pens on paper scrolling through the machine. But then, ninety minutes after sleep onset, there was a dramatic change; the pens moved vigorously and made considerable noise doing so. Steve's brain was very active, his breathing irregular, and his eyes were darting back and forth as if scanning the environment. Was he awake? Definitely not—at least not until Bill interrupted by asking, "What was going through your mind just now?" Steve groggily reported the first of his night's several episodes, this one featuring a baseball game. Then he rolled over and went back to sleep.

The rhythmic pattern of sleep and dreaming repeated itself every ninety minutes throughout the night. There were periods of movement and periods of quiescence, periods of dreaming and periods of total unawareness, as well as dramatic changes in body temperature, respiration, heart rate, and even, so I was told, genital activity. I had always regarded sleep as basically a dull wasteland of monotonous non-behavior, occasionally punctuated by a dream usually forgotten by breakfast time. How little I knew. How much I wanted to learn. I had no idea that the physiological and psychological architecture of the night was so complex.

In the weeks that followed, my mind filled with questions. What was the purpose of such varied sleep activity? Why did we need to sleep, and, if so, how much sleep did we need? What caused insomnia? How many sleep disorders were there? Could sleep problems be cured through medication or psychotherapy? Did lack of sleep cause illnesses such as hypertension and cancer? Did people gain or lose weight while they slept? Did sleep play a role in learning and memory? Did people need less sleep as they got older? Did women need more sleep than men? Were naps good for you? How could you overcome jetlag?

Bill Dement told me we didn't know most of the answers, but scientists were starting to develop research techniques that might provide some clues. He stimulated me to explore sleep and try to add my own contribution to the growing knowledge base regarding the third of our lives we spend (or should spend) sleeping. So I started to read the existing literature. I built a sleep lab at Cornell, made some films on sleep disorders, and began to write about what I had learned. I soon had plenty of company. The science of sleep grew from a discipline involving a handful of investigators in the 1970s to the now more than twenty thousand sleep researchers worldwide who are producing a prodigious body of scientific findings every year.

In my first few sleepless years as a teacher and researcher, I spent about forty-five minutes each semester discussing sleep in my classes. At first, there wasn't all that much to say beyond describing the stages of sleep and a few sleep disorders. I am now beginning my forty-seventh year at Cornell, where the 250-student class has grown over time to nearly 2,000, mostly sleep-deprived, students. Because of the proliferation of research findings, I now feel compelled to spend at least nine hours of the semester lecturing on the science of sleep.

At this point, I have had the pleasure of introducing more than sixty-five thousand Cornell undergraduates to everything from Freud's theory of dream interpretation to the physiological basis of sleep, lucid dreaming, sleep disorders, and the relationship between sleep and cognitive behavior, athletic performance, health, and longevity. Many of my students have taken my advice to value sleep and have noted significant improvement in their academic performance, social life, athletic prowess, and health. If students don't respond to my plea for getting more sleep, at least I build guilt in their tired minds and exhausted bodies.☺

I have a great deal of pleasure talking about sleep every week to newspaper and magazine editors. I get to appear frequently on national television programs such as NBC's *Today Show*, ABC's *World News*, *20/20*, and *Regis and Kelly*, and I have even spent time in bed talking with Katie Couric and Oprah—on national television in front of millions. We're trying to make sure the world is awakening to the fact that sleep is a necessity, not a luxury. It's no longer wise or healthy to be macho and get by on little sleep. It's downright dangerous.

Nearly every writer or broadcaster who interviews me ends the conversation with the same question: "Dr. Maas, how do you sleep?" I am no different from anybody else. I try to get eight hours on a regular sleep-wake schedule. But the demands of work, travel, and family sometimes interfere—and I feel lousy, drained, clumsy, and stupid. But as time goes by and my priorities change due to my knowledge about sleep and the wisdom that comes with experience and aging, I am definitely making progress—and I am able to *Sleep for Success!*

We are definitely beginning to make a difference. Attitudes about sleep are changing, albeit too slowly. My personal indication is that I, often with the assistance of Rebecca Robbins, Sharon Driscoll and Hannah Appelbaum, have been invited to give more than 70 lectures each year to Fortune 500 companies, educational institutions, associations, medical organizations, and professional sports franchises. A typical year would include clients such as: IBM, Eastman Kodak, Campbell's Soups, Pepsi Cola, Goldman Sachs, JP Morgan, the Young Presidents' Organization (YPO), the Naval War College, the American College of Facial and Plastic Surgeons, the United States Figure Skating Association, the NBA Orlando Magic, and the New York Jets.

One of the most exciting and rewarding experiences has been our involvement with prep schools, getting them to pay attention to sleep as a critical factor in academic success. I'll let Rebecca tell you about that in a moment.

So, where are we now, and what does the future hold? We have identified eighty-nine differentially diagnosable sleep disorders, and countless lives are being saved by doctor and patient education and through the use of effective medical and psychological therapies. We can provide good advice on sleep hygiene and how to minimize the effects of shift work and jetlag. We can design good bedroom environments. We can improve productivity and mental and athletic performance. But, we don't know the exact reasons as to why we need to sleep, other than to keep away feelings of sleepiness and to ensure good health. We have miles to go in convincing more people around the world that sleep is a necessity, not a luxury. There are still far too many sleep-related accidents, and far too many people suffer health issues due to lack of sleep. And the present global economy and its related stressors certainly aren't helping our ability to sleep long and deep.

I would hope that soon we will have medications that can give troubled sleepers a good night's sleep with minimal side effects. It might not be too long before we have a pill that attempts to significantly reduce our need for sleep, if not totally eliminate it. This would have a rather profound effect on work, social, and family life—can you imagine never having to go to sleep? But I predict that any such pill will have serious deleterious side effects. And, can you imagine life without the opportunity to enjoy restful, quiet hours in the cocoon of peaceful sleep?

Meanwhile, sweet REMs!

Rebecca Robbins

Before I began my research on sleep and the consequences of sleep deprivation, I did not have excellent sleep habits, to say the least. Between two swim practices a day and a rigorous academic schedule, I survived high school due to a steady infusion of caffeine. Getting me out of bed in the morning was a constant struggle, for which my wonderful mother deserves a medal.

In order to balance athletics, academics, and extracurriculars in my first year at Cornell, I fell into the same vicious cycle of late nights of studying, running up a never-ending coffee bill, and having an utterly irregular sleep schedule. This lifestyle seemed to be reinforced by my environment. The libraries were always packed in the evenings with students clutching a cup of coffee into the wee hours of the morning. Students constantly complained of how little sleep they'd had.

My mood deteriorated, academic performance plummeted, and desire to exercise, eat healthy food, and socialize diminished. I began to work with Dr. Maas and became aware that sleep deprivation was at the root of my problems. It took a while to break my previous habits; however, once I learned the necessity of getting my eight hours and all the strategies to do so, my academic performance, mood, and athletic ability all changed for the positive. I now have tremendous happiness and energy I never knew possible.

At about this time, my little brother was attending Deerfield Academy, a preparatory school long known for its achievement-oriented and, inadvertently, sleep-deprived and stressed students. Dr. Maas and I were invited to speak with the faculty and students on the facts about the relationship between sleep and academic performance. With the encouragement of the headmistress, Margarita Curtis, we proposed altering the school's schedule to allow for one extra hour of sleep. The faculty was not overly enthusiastic about our proposed changes, but they agreed to a trial semester. With a schedule that allowed for more sleep, the school witnessed improved academic performance across all grades, better mood, reduced illness, and greater success in athletics. The teachers were convinced that this was the way to go. As a result, we have been invited to initiate change at scores of educational institutions in the United States and Asia.

It's been exciting to carry our message to Fortune 500 companies, the Orlando Magic, and the New York Jets. In each case, our clients have experienced a significant improvement in performance as a result of being educated on the beneficial effects of valuing sleep. It's been tremendously rewarding to me to effect change, but I know we're only at the beginning of our mission to debunk the myth that it's macho to exist on little sleep.

In our twenty-four-hour society, I have seen how easy it is to fall into a downward spiral of overworking and under sleeping. Why succumb to this when a healthy, positive solution is at hand? If you value sleep and implement our strategies in your everyday life (make no mistake—it takes discipline), we guarantee you will have a happier, more productive, and healthier life ahead. Personally, paying attention to my sleep has quite literally changed my life. I hope the book you've just read will inspire you to *Sleep for Success!*

Appendix A

Sleep for Success Performance Log

Peak Performance Sleep Log
Copyright ©2010 Dr. James B. Maas

Every morning at breakfast fill out the chart for the previous day and night.
For example, on Monday morning you should complete the "Sunday" column.

Nights:	Sunday	Monday	Tuesday	Wednesday	Thursday	Friday	Saturday
What time did you turn your lights out?							
What time did you get up this morning?							
How many total hours did you sleep?							
How many times did you wake up during the night?							
Rate the quality of your sleep last night. 1 = terrible to 5 = great							
Did you avoid taking a nap yesterday?	Yes ☐ No ☐	Yes ☐ No ☐	Yes ☐ No ☐	Yes ☐ No ☐	Yes ☐ No ☐	Yes ☐ No ☐	Yes ☐ No ☐
Did you avoid caffeine after 6 PM?	Yes ☐ No ☐	Yes ☐ No ☐	Yes ☐ No ☐	Yes ☐ No ☐	Yes ☐ No ☐	Yes ☐ No ☐	Yes ☐ No ☐
Did you avoid alcohol after 6 PM?	Yes ☐ No ☐	Yes ☐ No ☐	Yes ☐ No ☐	Yes ☐ No ☐	Yes ☐ No ☐	Yes ☐ No ☐	Yes ☐ No ☐
Did you do anything to reduce stress yesterday?	Yes ☐ No ☐	Yes ☐ No ☐	Yes ☐ No ☐	Yes ☐ No ☐	Yes ☐ No ☐	Yes ☐ No ☐	Yes ☐ No ☐
Did you avoid sleeping medications?	Yes ☐ No ☐	Yes ☐ No ☐	Yes ☐ No ☐	Yes ☐ No ☐	Yes ☐ No ☐	Yes ☐ No ☐	Yes ☐ No ☐
Was your bedroom quiet, dark, and cool?	Yes ☐ No ☐	Yes ☐ No ☐	Yes ☐ No ☐	Yes ☐ No ☐	Yes ☐ No ☐	Yes ☐ No ☐	Yes ☐ No ☐
Did you do anything to relax before falling asleep?	Yes ☐ No ☐	Yes ☐ No ☐	Yes ☐ No ☐	Yes ☐ No ☐	Yes ☐ No ☐	Yes ☐ No ☐	Yes ☐ No ☐
Did you eat a balanced diet yesterday?	Yes ☐ No ☐	Yes ☐ No ☐	Yes ☐ No ☐	Yes ☐ No ☐	Yes ☐ No ☐	Yes ☐ No ☐	Yes ☐ No ☐
Did you exercise yesterday?	Yes ☐ No ☐	Yes ☐ No ☐	Yes ☐ No ☐	Yes ☐ No ☐	Yes ☐ No ☐	Yes ☐ No ☐	Yes ☐ No ☐
How alert and energetic did you feel during the day? 1 = sleepy, tired to 5 = fully alert, energetic							

How are you doing? To be prepared for peak performance (5's in the last row):
1. You should be getting close to eight hours of sleep each night.
2. Your sleep and wake times should not change between weekdays and weekends.
3. Your sleep should be continuous, not fragmented.
4. Your sleep should be restful.
5. The answers to all the yes-or-no questions should be yes.

Peak Performance Sleep Log
Copyright ©2010 Dr. James B. Maas

Week Two

Every morning at breakfast fill out the chart for the previous day and night. For example, on Monday morning you should complete the "Sunday" column.

Nights:	Sunday	Monday	Tuesday	Wednesday	Thursday	Friday	Saturday
What time did you turn your lights out?							
What time did you get up this morning?							
How many total hours did you sleep?							
How many times did you wake up during the night?							
Rate the quality of your sleep last night. 1 = terrible to 5 = great							
Did you avoid taking a nap yesterday?	Yes ☐ No ☐	Yes ☐ No ☐	Yes ☐ No ☐	Yes ☐ No ☐	Yes ☐ No ☐	Yes ☐ No ☐	Yes ☐ No ☐
Did you avoid caffeine after 6 PM?	Yes ☐ No ☐	Yes ☐ No ☐	Yes ☐ No ☐	Yes ☐ No ☐	Yes ☐ No ☐	Yes ☐ No ☐	Yes ☐ No ☐
Did you avoid alcohol after 6 PM?	Yes ☐ No ☐	Yes ☐ No ☐	Yes ☐ No ☐	Yes ☐ No ☐	Yes ☐ No ☐	Yes ☐ No ☐	Yes ☐ No ☐
Did you do anything to reduce stress yesterday?	Yes ☐ No ☐	Yes ☐ No ☐	Yes ☐ No ☐	Yes ☐ No ☐	Yes ☐ No ☐	Yes ☐ No ☐	Yes ☐ No ☐
Did you avoid sleeping medications?	Yes ☐ No ☐	Yes ☐ No ☐	Yes ☐ No ☐	Yes ☐ No ☐	Yes ☐ No ☐	Yes ☐ No ☐	Yes ☐ No ☐
Was your bedroom quiet, dark, and cool?	Yes ☐ No ☐	Yes ☐ No ☐	Yes ☐ No ☐	Yes ☐ No ☐	Yes ☐ No ☐	Yes ☐ No ☐	Yes ☐ No ☐
Did you do anything to relax before falling asleep?	Yes ☐ No ☐	Yes ☐ No ☐	Yes ☐ No ☐	Yes ☐ No ☐	Yes ☐ No ☐	Yes ☐ No ☐	Yes ☐ No ☐
Did you eat a balanced diet yesterday?	Yes ☐ No ☐	Yes ☐ No ☐	Yes ☐ No ☐	Yes ☐ No ☐	Yes ☐ No ☐	Yes ☐ No ☐	Yes ☐ No ☐
Did you exercise yesterday?	Yes ☐ No ☐	Yes ☐ No ☐	Yes ☐ No ☐	Yes ☐ No ☐	Yes ☐ No ☐	Yes ☐ No ☐	Yes ☐ No ☐
How alert and energetic did you feel during the day? 1 = sleepy, tired to 5 = fully alert, energetic							

How are you doing? To be prepared for peak performance (5's in the last row):

1. You should be getting close to eight hours of sleep each night.
2. Your sleep and wake times should not change between weekdays and weekends.
3. Your sleep should be continuous, not fragmented.
4. Your sleep should be restful.
5. The answers to all the yes-or-no questions should be yes.

Peak Performance Sleep Log
Copyright ©2010 Dr. James B. Maas

Every morning at breakfast fill out the chart for the previous day and night.
For example, on Monday morning you should complete the "Sunday" column.

Nights:	Sunday	Monday	Tuesday	Wednesday	Thursday	Friday	Saturday
What time did you turn your lights out?							
What time did you get up this morning?							
How many total hours did you sleep?							
How many times did you wake up during the night?							
Rate the quality of your sleep last night. 1 = terrible to 5 = great							
Did you avoid taking a nap yesterday?	Yes ☐ No ☐	Yes ☐ No ☐	Yes ☐ No ☐	Yes ☐ No ☐	Yes ☐ No ☐	Yes ☐ No ☐	Yes ☐ No ☐
Did you avoid caffeine after 6 PM?	Yes ☐ No ☐	Yes ☐ No ☐	Yes ☐ No ☐	Yes ☐ No ☐	Yes ☐ No ☐	Yes ☐ No ☐	Yes ☐ No ☐
Did you avoid alcohol after 6 PM?	Yes ☐ No ☐	Yes ☐ No ☐	Yes ☐ No ☐	Yes ☐ No ☐	Yes ☐ No ☐	Yes ☐ No ☐	Yes ☐ No ☐
Did you do anything to reduce stress yesterday?	Yes ☐ No ☐	Yes ☐ No ☐	Yes ☐ No ☐	Yes ☐ No ☐	Yes ☐ No ☐	Yes ☐ No ☐	Yes ☐ No ☐
Did you avoid sleeping medications?	Yes ☐ No ☐	Yes ☐ No ☐	Yes ☐ No ☐	Yes ☐ No ☐	Yes ☐ No ☐	Yes ☐ No ☐	Yes ☐ No ☐
Was your bedroom quiet, dark, and cool?	Yes ☐ No ☐	Yes ☐ No ☐	Yes ☐ No ☐	Yes ☐ No ☐	Yes ☐ No ☐	Yes ☐ No ☐	Yes ☐ No ☐
Did you do anything to relax before falling asleep?	Yes ☐ No ☐	Yes ☐ No ☐	Yes ☐ No ☐	Yes ☐ No ☐	Yes ☐ No ☐	Yes ☐ No ☐	Yes ☐ No ☐
Did you eat a balanced diet yesterday?	Yes ☐ No ☐	Yes ☐ No ☐	Yes ☐ No ☐	Yes ☐ No ☐	Yes ☐ No ☐	Yes ☐ No ☐	Yes ☐ No ☐
Did you exercise yesterday?	Yes ☐ No ☐	Yes ☐ No ☐	Yes ☐ No ☐	Yes ☐ No ☐	Yes ☐ No ☐	Yes ☐ No ☐	Yes ☐ No ☐
How alert and energetic did you feel during the day? 1 = sleepy, tired to 5 = fully alert, energetic							

How are you doing? To be prepared for peak performance (5's in the last row):
1. You should be getting close to eight hours of sleep each night.
2. Your sleep and wake times should not change between weekdays and weekends.
3. Your sleep should be continuous, not fragmented.
4. Your sleep should be restful.
5. The answers to all the yes-or-no questions should be yes.

Peak Performance Sleep Log
Copyright ©2010 Dr. James B. Maas

Every morning at breakfast fill out the chart for the previous day and night.
For example, on Monday morning you should complete the "Sunday" column.

Week Four

Nights:	Sunday	Monday	Tuesday	Wednesday	Thursday	Friday	Saturday
What time did you turn your lights out?							
What time did you get up this morning?							
How many total hours did you sleep?							
How many times did you wake up during the night?							
Rate the quality of your sleep last night. 1 = terrible to 5 = great							
Did you avoid taking a nap yesterday?	Yes ☐ No ☐	Yes ☐ No☐	Yes ☐ No ☐	Yes ☐ No ☐	Yes ☐ No ☐	Yes ☐ No ☐	Yes ☐ No ☐
Did you avoid caffeine after 6 PM?	Yes ☐ No ☐	Yes ☐ No ☐	Yes ☐ No ☐	Yes ☐ No ☐	Yes ☐ No ☐	Yes ☐ No ☐	Yes ☐ No ☐
Did you avoid alcohol after 6 PM?	Yes ☐ No ☐	Yes ☐ No ☐	Yes ☐ No ☐	Yes ☐ No ☐	Yes ☐ No ☐	Yes ☐ No ☐	Yes ☐ No☐
Did you do anything to reduce stress yesterday?	Yes ☐ No ☐	Yes ☐ No ☐	Yes ☐ No ☐	Yes ☐ No ☐	Yes ☐ No ☐	Yes ☐ No ☐	Yes ☐ No ☐
Did you avoid sleeping medications?	Yes ☐ No ☐	Yes ☐ No ☐	Yes ☐ No ☐	Yes ☐ No ☐	Yes ☐ No ☐	Yes ☐ No ☐	Yes ☐ No ☐
Was your bedroom quiet, dark, and cool?	Yes ☐ No ☐	Yes ☐ No ☐	Yes ☐ No ☐	Yes ☐ No ☐	Yes ☐ No ☐	Yes ☐ No ☐	Yes ☐ No ☐
Did you do anything to relax before falling asleep?	Yes ☐ No ☐	Yes ☐ No ☐	Yes ☐ No ☐	Yes ☐ No ☐	Yes ☐ No ☐	Yes ☐ No ☐	Yes ☐ No ☐
Did you eat a balanced diet yesterday?	Yes ☐ No ☐	Yes ☐ No ☐	Yes ☐ No ☐	Yes ☐ No ☐	Yes ☐ No ☐	Yes ☐ No ☐	Yes ☐ No ☐
Did you exercise yesterday?	Yes ☐ No ☐	Yes ☐ No ☐	Yes ☐ No ☐	Yes ☐ No ☐	Yes ☐ No ☐	Yes ☐ No ☐	Yes ☐ No ☐
How alert and energetic did you feel during the day? 1 = sleepy, tired to 5 = fully alert, energetic							

How are you doing? To be prepared for peak performance (5's in the last row):
1. You should be getting close to eight hours of sleep each night.
2. Your sleep and wake times should not change between weekdays and weekends.
3. Your sleep should be continuous, not fragmented.
4. Your sleep should be restful.
5. The answers to all the yes-or-no questions should be yes.

APPENDIX B

Suggested Readings and Videotapes on Sleep

Part One: Everything You Must Know About Sleep but Are Too Tired to Ask

Caldwell, Paul. *Sleep*. Toronto, Canada: Key Porter Books Limited, 1995. General information on sleep featuring side bars, case studies and diagrams.

Carskadon, Mary A. *The Encyclopedia of Sleep and Dreaming*. New York: MacMillan, 1993. Covers in detail absolutely everything you have ever wanted to know about sleep or dreams.

Dement, William C. *The Promise of Sleep*. New York: Random House, 1999. Explores the vital connections between health, happiness, and a good night's sleep.

Hobson, J. Allan. *Sleep*. New York: Freeman & Co., 1989. A classic that recounts the science of sleep and dreams for the layperson, providing a coherent view of modern sleep research. Uncovers the cellular and molecular mechanisms by which the brain regulates sleeping behavior.

Mitler, Elizabeth A., and Merrill M. Mitler. *101 Questions About Sleep and Dreams*. Del Mar, Calif.: Wakefulness-Sleep Education and Research Foundation, 1996. Provides short, accurate answers to some of the most commonly asked questions.

Part Two: New Discoveries in the Science of Sleep

Cartwright, Rosalind. *The Twenty-Four Hour Mind*. New York: Oxford University Press, 2010. Looks at the role of sleep and dreaming in our emotional lives.

Hobson, Allan J. *The Dreaming Brain*. New York: Basic Books, 1988. A research-based reference book on the history of dreams and dream interpretation.

Part Three: A New Look on How to Get a Great Eight Hours of Sleep!

Anthony, William A. *The Art of Napping*. Burdett, NY: Larson Publications, 1997. A lighthearted guide to getting the most out of a nap.

Breus, Michael. *Good Night*. New York: Penguin Books Ltd., 2006. Outlines how to identify sleep issues, and what you can do about it.

Dinges, David and Roger Broughton. *Sleep and Alertness: Chronological, Behavioral and Medical Aspects of Napping*. New York: Raven, 1990. A bible of research on napping.

Epstein, Lawrence J. *A Good Night's Sleep*. New York: McGraw-Hill, 2007. Explains health benefits of sleep and identifies signs of sleep problems, and advice.

Inlander, Charles B. and Cynthia K. Moran. *67 Ways to Good Sleep*. New York: Ballantine Books, 1995. Includes ways to maximize sleep in relation with diet, sleep environment, sleeping pills, and sleep disorders.

Kavey, Neil B. *50 Ways to Sleep Better*. Lincolnwood, Ill.: Publications International Ltd., 1996. Handy hints for a restful night.

Kryger, Meir. *A Good Night's Sleep*. New York: Metro Books, 2009. The National Sleep Foundation's guide to sleeping well.

Mednick, Sara C. *Take a Nap! Change Your Life*. New York: Workman Publishing Co., 2006. Lessons on how to take the ultimate nap.

Part Four: Helpful Solutions to Common Sleep Challenges

Carskadon, Mary A. *Adolescent Sleep Patterns: Biological, Social, and Psychological Influences*. Cambridge, UK: Cambridge University Press, 2002. Reveals the effects of environmental factors such as work and school schedule on adolescent sleep.

Coren, Stanley. *Sleep Thieves: An Eye-opening Exploration into the Science & Mysteries of Sleep*. New York: Free Press, 1996. Chronicles the need to place more importance on the role of sleep in our society.

Dotto, Lydia. *Losing Sleep*. NY: William Morrow, 1990. The best overview of sleep studies related to jobs and performance.

Ferber, Richard. *Solve Your Child's Sleep Problems*. New York: Simon & Schuster, 1985. For parents whose children are experiencing sleep problems.

Ferber, Richard and Meir Kryger. *Principles and Practices of Sleep Medicine in the Child*. New York: Saunders, 1995. A medical textbook that deals with the troubled sleep of children.

Maas, James B., Rebecca S. Robbins, Rebecca G. Fortgang, and Sharon R. Driscoll. *Adolescent Sleep*. Encyclopedia of Adolescence. Cambridge, UK: Elsevier, 2011. Overview on all issues related to adolescents and sleep.

Moore-Ede, Martin. *The Twenty-Four-Hour Society*. New York: Addison Wesley, 1993.Understanding human limits in a world that never stops.

Morgan, Kevin. *Sleep and Aging: A Research-Based Guide to Sleep in Later Life*. Baltimore, MD: John Hopkins University Press, 1987.

Oren, Dan. A. et al. *How to Beat Jet Lag*. New York: Henry Holt, 1993. Step-by-step instructions in conquering jet lag, and handling red-eye flights.

Owens, Judy A. and Jodi A. Mindell. *Take Charge of Your Child's Sleep*. New York: Marlowe and Co., 2005. The all-in-one resource for solving sleep problems in kids and teens.

Ricci, Judith A., Elsbeth Chee, Amy L. Lorandeau, and Jan Berger. *Fatigue in the U.S. Workforce: Prevalence and Implications for Lost Productive Work Time*. Journal of Occupational and Environmental Medicine, 2007.

Walsleben, Joyce and Rita Baron-Faust. *A Woman's Guide to Sleep*. New York: Crown Publishers, 2000. Guaranteed solutions for a good night's rest.

Wolfson, Amy. *The Woman's Book of Sleep.* Oakland, Calif.: New Harbinger Publications, 2001. A comprehensive guide on women's sleep issues.

Part Five: An Up-to-Date Look at Sleep Disorders and Their Treatment

Foldvary-Schaefer, Nancy. *The Cleveland Clinic Guide to Sleep Disorders.* New York: Kaplan, 2009. Discover how to recognize when you have a sleep disorder, and improve your sleep habits.

Ford, Norman. *The Sleep R$_x$. Englewood Cliffs, NJ: Prentice Hall, 1994.* Details the architecture of a good-nights sleep, self-diagnosis of insomnia, and suggested cures.

Fritz, Roger. *Sleep Disorders: America's Hidden Nightmare.* Naperville, Ill.: National Sleep Alert, Inc., 1993. A review of sleep deprivation and sleep disorders.

Hauri, Peter and Shirley Linde. *No More Sleepless Nights.* New York: John Wiley & Sons, Inc., 1990. An excellent guide for adults with sleep problems.

Kryger, Meir H., Thomas Roth, and William C. Dement. *Principles and Practices of Sleep Medicine.* New York: Saunders, 1994. A medical textbook outlining methods of the various treatments used to cure sleep disorders.

Lavie, Peretz. *The Enchanted World of Sleep.* New Haven: Yale University Press, 1996. A very readable survey of sleep research and sleep medicine.

Morin, Charles M. *Insomnia: Psychological Assessment and Management.* New York: The Guilford Press, 1993. Designed as a hands-on resource for health professionals.

Neubauer, David. *Understanding Sleeplessness.* Baltimore, MD: John Hopkins University Press, 2003.

Pascualy, Ralph A. and Sally Warren Soest. *Snoring and Sleep Apnea: Personal and Family Guide to Diagnosis and Treatment.* New York:

Raven Press, 1994. Details on sleep apnea, as well as some handy hints about stopping snorers.

Regestein, Quentin R., et al., eds. *Sleep: Problems and Solutions.* Mount Vernon, NY: Consumer Union Report Books, 1990.

Schneck, Carlos. *Sleep: The Mysteries, The Problems, and The Solutions.* New York: Avery, 2007. The latest scientific discoveries in understanding and treating sleep disorders.

Shapiro, Colin. M. *Conquering Insomnia: An Illustrated Guide to Understanding Sleep and a Manual for Overcoming Sleep Disruption.* Hamilton, Ont.: Empowering Press, 1994.

Thorpy, Michal and Jan Yager. *The Encyclopedia of Sleep and Sleep Disorders.* New York: Facts of File Inc., 2001. Examines and discusses the important terms, conditions, remedies, and advances made in sleep research and sleep-disorder treatment.

Utley, Margaret Jones. *Narcolepsy: A Funny Disorder That's No Laughing Matter.* A great source for information on narcolepsy that is easy to read and includes the author's own experiences with the disease. To order, contact M.J. Utley, PO Box 1923, DeSoto, TX 75123-1923.

Zammit, Gary. *Good Nights.* Kansas City, MO: Andrews and McMeel, 1997. How to stop sleep deprivation, overcome insomnia, and get the sleep you need.

For further information about sleep and sleep disorders, contact:
National Sleep Foundation, 1522 K Street NW, Suite 500, Washington, DC 20005

Videotapes on Sleep

Maas, James B. and David H. Gluck. "Keep Us Awake." Ithaca, NY: Cornell University Psychology Film Unit, 1978. A documentary film on the symptoms, causes, and treatment of narcolepsy.

Maas, James B. and David H. Gluck. "When Nights are Longest." Ithaca, NY: Cornell University Psychology Film Unit, 1983. A documentary on the symptoms, causes, and cures for the various syndromes that constitute the sleep disorder of insomnia.

Maas, James B. "Sleep Alert." Ithaca, NY: Cornell University Psychology Film Unit, 1993. A PBS nationwide prime-time special on the problem of sleep deprivation in America.

Maas, James B. "Asleep in the Fast Lane: Our 24-Hour Society." Ithaca, NY: Cornell University Psychology Film Unit, 1997. A documentary on how lack of sleep causes accidents and poor performance in our fast-paced society.

Maas, James B. "Who Needs Sleep?" Ithaca, NY: Cornell University Psychology Film Unit, 2006. An educational video (shot in MTV style) for high school students needing information on the deleterious consequences of sleep deprivation, and the rules of good sleep hygiene.

Stuart, Melvin. "The Mystery of Sleep." Los Angeles, Calif.: Mel Stuart Productions, 2010. Contact Mel Stuart Productions by phone at: 213-785-9080, or by mail at: 1551 South Robertson Blvd., Los Angeles, CA 90035

(All of the videotapes produced by Prof. Maas are available from Dr. James B. Maas, 211C Uris Hall, Department of Psychology, Cornell University, Ithaca, New York, 14853. 607-255-6266)

APPENDIX C

Internet Resources

The Sleep Well:
http://www-leland.stanford.edu/~dement/

A tremendous source of up-to-date information on all aspects of sleep. From Stanford University, a major center for sleep research. Includes a calendar of sleep-related events, an extensive bibliography and the addresses of sleep disorders associations and help groups.

The Sleepnet Home Page:
http://www.sleepnet.com/

Everything you want to know about sleep but are too tired to ask. Provides some startling statistics as well as more than 130 rated **hot links** to other sleep websites.

National Sleep Foundation:
http://www.sleepfoundation.org/

This is a direct link to the best known non-profit foundation for sleep. Here you can get the answers to questions you have concerning everything from children and sleep to adolescent sleep and changing school start times to napping, jet lag, sleep disorders and sleep aids.

Access to Sleep and Psychology:
http://health.yahoo.net/channel/sleep-disorders.html

An academic science site: Basic "how to" and "self-help" regarding sleep research and psychology. Includes abstracts on Melatonin and sleep, health, and development.

NIH Guide to Healthy Sleep:
http://www.nhlbi.nih.gov/health/public/sleep/healthy_sleep.pdf

This patient and public booklet provides the latest science-based information about Sleep, common sleep myths and practical tips for getting adequate sleep, coping with jet lag and nighttime shift work and avoiding dangerous drowsy driving.

The Sleep Medicine Home Page:
http://www.cloud9.net/~thorpy/

This website provides links to information sites concerning virtually every sleep disorder, and to sleep physicians, listings of Sleep Disorder

Centers, Research Centers, Sleep-related Foundations, and Professional Associations.

The School of Sleep Medicine:
http://www.sleepedu.net/

The School of Sleep Medicine (SSM) was founded to provide high quality education for the medical community worldwide. Its purpose is to increase awareness among physicians and other health care professionals of the nature and treatment of sleep disorders.

Narcolepsy:
http://med.stanford.edu/school/Psychiatry/narcolepsy/

The Stanford University Center for Narcolepsy home page. Interests of the research center range from finding better pharmacological treatments for human patients to isolating the genes for narcolepsy.

Which CPAP Machine is Best For You?:
http://www.mayoclinic.com/health/cpap-masks/SL00018.

This slide show from sleep experts at the Mayo Clinic will help Sleep Apnea patients fit their CPAP machine correctly.

National Health Institute Guide on Sleep Apnea:
http://newsinhealth.nih.gov/2007/April/docs/01features_02.htm

Guide for understanding the disorder and its symptoms, causes and treatment.

Sleep and Dreams:
http://www.asdreams.org/index.htm
The International Association for the Study of Dreams is a non-profit, international, multidisciplinary organization dedicated to the pure and applied investigation of dreams and dreaming.

Phantom Sleep Page:
http://www.newtechpub.com/phantom/

A site for those who think they may be suffering from sleep apnea. Includes information on snoring and other sleep problems as well as a free self-scoring sleep apnea quiz.

Sleep for Success, LLC.

Life changing keynote presentations, training programs and seminars

Almost everybody is sleep deprived. To be a peak performer you need to be fully alert, dynamic, energetic, in a good mood, and cognitively sharp. This is only possible through quality sleep.

Our multi-media presentations, extremely popular with corporations, educational institutions, athletic franchises and general audiences, focus on giving you the tools to radically jumpstart your life. We will answer questions such as:

- What are the consequences of sleep deprivation on thinking, performance, health, and lifespan?
- What are the four golden rules and ten sleep strategies that will assure you a great night's sleep and a better tomorrow?
- What are the five stages of nocturnal sleep and why are they essential for maximum functioning?
- How can you reduce travel fatigue?
- How can you increase your athletic performance overnight?
- Do you need less sleep as you get older?
- Can you learn while you sleep?
- Can napping improve cognitive abilities?
- How do you choose a great pillow and mattress?
- What causes insomnia and how can it be overcome?

The information provided will increase your daytime alertness, psychological mood, productivity, creativity, and quality of life. Our programs will show you highly specific behaviors and routines that will enhance your life immediately. The Sleep for Success training module can be delivered in a variety of ways, and customized to fit your organization's specific needs.

241

Dr. James B. Maas is one of the world's most noted award-winning lecturers. He has taught more than 65,000 university students in his 47 years on the Cornell University faculty. Sleep for Success consultants Rebecca S. Robbins and Sharon R. Driscoll, experts in sleep and in communications, have both presented highly successful programs on sleep to scores of corporations and educational institutions.

For more information on Sleep for Success Presentations, contact Dr. James B. Maas at maas.james@gmail.com and visit www.sleepforsuccess.info or www.powersleep.com

To order *Sleep for Success!* pillows and other bedding products designed to promote better sleep, go to http://www.ufandd.com/ on the internet.